Myelodysplastic Syndromes

Editor

ALEXA J. SIDDON

CLINICS IN LABORATORY MEDICINE

www.labmed.theclinics.com

Consulting Editor
MILENKO JOVAN TANASIJEVIC

December 2023 • Volume 43 • Number 4

ELSEVIER

1600 John F. Kennedy Boulevard • Suite 1800 • Philadelphia, Pennsylvania, 19103-2899

http://www.theclinics.com

CLINICS IN LABORATORY MEDICINE Volume 43, Number 4
December 2023 ISSN 0272-2712, ISBN-13: 978-0-443-12999-5

Editor: Taylor Hayes
Developmental Editor: Akshay Samson

Reprints. For copies of 100 or more, of articles in this publication, please contact the Commercial Reprints Department, Elsevier Inc., 360 Park Avenue South, New York, New York 10010-1710. Tel. 212-633-3874, Fax: 212-633-3820, E-mail: reprints@elsevier.com.

Clinics in Laboratory Medicine (ISSN 0272-2712) is published quarterly by Elsevier Inc., 360 Park Avenue South, New York, NY 10010-1710. Months of issue are March, June, September, and December. Business and Editorial offices: 1600 John F. Kennedy Blvd., Suite 1800, Philadelphia, PA 19103-2899. Periodicals postage paid at NewYork, NY and additional mailing offices. Subscription prices are $291.00 per year (US individuals), $657.00 per year (US institutions), $100.00 per year (US students), $374.00 per year (Canadian individuals), $798.00 per year (Canadian institutions), $100.00 per year (Canadian students), $416.00 per year (international individuals), $798.00 per year (international institutions), $185.00 (international students). Foreign air speed delivery is included in all Clinics subscription prices. All prices are subject to change without notice. POSTMASTER: Send address changes to *Clinics in Laboratory Medicine*, Elsevier Health Sciences Division, Subscription Customer Service, 3251 Riverport Lane, Maryland Heights, MO 63043. **Customer Service: 1-800-654-2452 (US). From outside of the US and Canada, call 1-314-447-8871. Fax: 1-314-447-8029. E-mail: journalscustomerservice-usa@elsevier.com (for print support) or journalsonlinesupport-usa@elsevier.com (for online support).**

Clinics in Laboratory Medicine is covered in *EMBASE/Exerpta Medica, MEDLINE/PubMed (Index Medicus), Cinahl, Current Contents/Clinical Medicine, BIOSIS* and *ISI/BIOMED*.

Contributors

CONSULTING EDITOR

MILENKO JOVAN TANASIJEVIC, MD, MBA
Vice Chair for Clinical Pathology and Quality, Department of Pathology, Director of Clinical Laboratories, Brigham and Women's Hospital, Dana-Farber Cancer Institute, Associate Professor of Pathology, Harvard Medical School, Boston, Massachusetts, USA

EDITOR

ALEXA J. SIDDON, MD
Associate Professor, Department of Laboratory Medicine and Pathology, Yale School of Medicine, New Haven, Connecticut, USA

AUTHORS

SANDRA D. BOHLING, MD
Clinical Assistant Professor, Associate Director, Hematopathology, Department of Laboratories, Seattle Children's Hospital, Clinical Assistant Professor, Department of Laboratory Medicine and Pathology, University of Washington Medical Center, Seattle, Washington, USA

KATHERINE R. CALVO, MD, PhD
Senior Research Physician and Director of Automated Hematology, Hematology Section, Department of Laboratory Medicine, Clinical Center, Myeloid Malignancies Program, National Institutes of Health, Bethesda, Maryland, USA

XUEYAN CHEN, MD, PhD
Associate Professor, Director, Developmental Hematopathology, Translational Science and Therapeutics Division, Fred Hutch Cancer Center, Department of Laboratory Medicine and Pathology, University of Washington, Seattle, Washington, USA

SINDHU CHERIAN, MD
Associate Director Hematopathology Laboratory, Department of Laboratory Medicine and Pathology, University of Washington, Seattle, Washington, USA

KAREN M. CHISHOLM, MD, PhD
Medical Director, Hematopathology, Department of Laboratories, Seattle Children's Hospital, Associate Professor, Department of Laboratory Medicine and Pathology, University of Washington Medical Center, Seattle, Washington, USA

KELLY E. CRAVEN, MD, PhD
Molecular Genetic Pathology Fellow, Department of Pathology and Laboratory Medicine, Memorial Sloan Kettering Cancer Center, New York, New York, USA

MARK D. EWALT, MD
Associate Attending, Molecular Genetic Pathology Fellow, Department of Pathology and Laboratory Medicine, Memorial Sloan Kettering Cancer Center, New York, New York, USA

DAVID C. GAJZER, MD
Department of Laboratory Medicine and Pathology, University of Washington, Seattle, Washington, USA

JULIANA GUARENTE, MD
Assistant Professor, Department of Pathology and Genomic Medicine, Assistant Director of Transfusion Medicine, Associate Director, Pathology Residency Program, Thomas Jefferson University Hospital, Philadelphia, Pennsylvania, USA

ROBERT P. HASSERJIAN, MD
Professor of Pathology, Director, Hematopathology Fellowship, Associate Director for Recruitment, Pathology Residency, Department of Pathology, Massachusetts General Hospital, Boston, Massachusetts, USA

ULRIKA JOHANSSON, PhD
Lead Scientist, SI-HMDS, University Hospitals Bristol and Weston NHS Foundation Trust, Bristol, United Kingdom

ADELAIDE KWON, MD
Resident, Department of Pathology, The University of Texas Southwestern Medical Center, Dallas, Texas, USA

YAZAN F. MADANAT, MD
Eugene P. Frenkel M.D. Scholar in Clinical Medicine, Division of Hematology and Medical Oncology, Harold C. Simmons Comprehensive Cancer Center, The University of Texas Southwestern Medical Center, Dallas, Texas, USA

HADRIAN MENDOZA, MD
Resident Physician, Department of Internal Medicine, Yale School of Medicine, New Haven, Connecticut, USA

IFEYINWA E. OBIORAH, MD, PhD
Assistant Professor, Department of Pathology, Division of Hematopathology, University of Virginia Health, Charlottesville, Virginia, USA

ALEXA J. SIDDON, MD
Associate Professor, Department of Laboratory Medicine and Pathology, Yale School of Medicine, New Haven, Connecticut, USA

CHRISTOPHER TORMEY, MD
Professor of Laboratory Medicine, Director, Transfusion Medicine Services, Director, Department of Laboratory Medicine, Transfusion Medicine Fellowship, Yale School of Medicine, Yale New Haven Hospital, New Haven, Connecticut, USA

KALPANA D. UPADHYAYA, PhD
Assistant Professor, Hematology Section, Department of Laboratory Medicine, Clinical Center, National Institutes of Health, Bethesda, Maryland, USA

OLGA K. WEINBERG, MD
Associate Professor, Department of Pathology, The University of Texas Southwestern Medical Center, BioCenter, Dallas, Texas, USA

CECILIA C.S. YEUNG, MD
Associate Professor, University of Washington, Fred Hutch Cancer Center, Seattle, Washington, USA

LISA D. YUEN, MD, PhD
Hematopathology Fellow, Department of Pathology, WRN 2, Massachusetts General Hospital, Boston, Massachusetts, USA

AMER M. ZEIDAN, MBBS
Associate Professor, Section of Hematology, Department of Internal Medicine, Yale Cancer Center, Smilow Cancer Center, Yale University, New Haven, Connecticut, USA

Contents

Myelodysplastic syndromes/neoplasms (MDS) are a heterogeneous class of hematopoietic stem cell neoplasms characterized by ineffective hematopoiesis leading to peripheral cytopenias. This group of diseases is typically diagnosed using a combination of clinical, morphologic, and genetic criteria. Many studies have described the value of multiparametric flow cytometry (MFC) in the diagnosis, classification, and prognostication of MDS. This review summarizes the approach to MDS diagnosis and immunophenotypic characterization using MFC and describes the current state while highlighting future opportunities and potential pitfalls.

Sequencing technology, particularly next-generation sequencing, has highlighted the importance of gene mutations in myelodysplastic syndromes (MDS). Mutations affecting DNA methylation, chromatin modification, RNA splicing, cohesin complex, and other pathways are present in most MDS cases and often have prognostic and clinical implications. Updated international diagnostic guidelines as well as the new International Prognostic Scoring System-Molecular incorporate molecular data into the diagnosis and prognostication of MDS. With whole-genome sequencing predicted to become the future standard of genetic evaluation, it is likely that MDS diagnosis and management will become increasingly personalized based on an individual's clinical and genomic profile.

Premalignant clonal hematopoiesis is the presence of somatic alterations in the blood of otherwise healthy individuals. Although the condition is not considered as a cancer, it carries an increased risk of developing a hematologic malignancy, particularly in those with large neoplastic clones, multiple pathogenic mutations, and high-risk mutations. In addition to the increased risk of malignancy, clonal hematopoiesis carries a markedly increased risk of cardiovascular events and death. Appropriate identification of this entity is critical to mitigate cardiovascular risk factors and ensure appropriate monitoring for the emergence of blood cancer.

Morphologic characterization remains a cornerstone in the diagnosis and classification of myelodysplastic syndromes (MDS) in the updated International Consensus Classification (ICC) and 5th edition World Health Organization Classification of Myeloid Neoplasms (Arber, Orazi, & Hasserjian, 2022; Khoury & Solary, 2022). The presence of dysplasia is one of the key diagnostic criteria required for establishing a diagnosis of MDS, and the percentage of myeloblasts in the blood and bone marrow impacts both disease classification and prognostication. Morphologic features also aid in distinguishing MDS from a myriad of other myeloid neoplasms and non-neoplastic mimics. Additional key morphologic features that should be recorded in any MDS case are the bone marrow cellularity and the degree of reticulin fibrosis. In this review, the morphologic assessment of the bone marrow biopsy, bone marrow aspirate, and peripheral blood smear as it pertains to the diagnosis and up-to-date classification of MDS will be described. The implications of the findings on classification and prognosis will also be discussed.

Myelodysplastic neoplasm with low blasts and *SF3B1* mutation (MDS-LB-*SF3B1*) has undergone significant classification changes in the past year with the publication of the 5th edition of the World Health Organization Classification of Tumors of Haematopoietic and Lymphoid Tissues and the International Consensus Classification. This article reviews the basic biology of *SF3B1*, iron metabolism, and dysfunction that leads to the formation of ring sideroblasts. It highlights neoplastic and non-neoplastic considerations to the differential diagnoses. Finally, a review on the evolution of the prognostic scoring system and treatment regimens that are available to patients with a diagnosis of MDS is presented.

The genetic underpinnings of myeloid neoplasms are becoming increasingly well understood. The accessibility to sequencing technology, in particular next-generation sequencing (NGS), has highlighted the importance of gene mutations in myelodysplastic syndromes (MDS) in conjunction with traditional cytogenetics. With the relatively recent influx of molecular information to complement known cytogenetic abnormalities, the diagnosis, classification, and prognosis of MDS and acute myeloid leukemia (AML) have been increasingly refined, which has also led to therapeutic advancements. It has been shown that *TP53* mutations have a significant impact in cases of MDS, as well as AML, and have led to *TP53*-defined myeloid disease. *TP53* mutations are also now incorporated into prognostic scoring systems, as patients have been shown to have aggressive disease and poor outcomes. With the increased understanding of the importance of *TP53* disruption in myeloid neoplasia, it is likely that the critical role of *TP53* will continue to be highlighted by an individual's disease classification and personalized therapeutic management.

Molecular and sequencing advances have led to substantial breakthroughs in the discovery of new genes and inherited mutations associated with increased risk of developing myeloid malignancies. Many of the same germline mutated genes are also drivers of malignancy in sporadic cancer. Recognition of myeloid malignancy associated with germline mutations is essential for proper therapy, disease surveillance, informing related donor selection for hematopoietic stem cell transplantation, and genetic counseling of the patient and affected family members. Some germline mutations are associated with syndromic features that precede the development of malignancy; however, penetrance may be highly variable leading to masking of the syndromic phenotype and/or inherited etiology.

Myelodysplastic syndrome (MDS) in children is rare, accounting for < 5% of all childhood hematologic malignancies. With the advent of next-generation sequencing, the etiology of many childhood MDS (cMDS) cases has been elucidated with the finding of predisposing germline mutations in one-quarter to one-third of cases; somatic mutations have also been identified, indicating that cMDS is different than adult MDS. Herein, cMDS classification schema, clinical presentation, laboratory values, bone marrow histology, differential diagnostic considerations, and the recent molecular findings of cMDS are described.

Myelodysplastic syndromes (MDS) are a group of myeloid neoplasms characterized by clonal hematopoiesis and abnormal maturation of hematopoietic cells, resulting in cytopenias. The transformation of MDS to acute myeloid leukemia (AML) reflects a progressive increase in blasts due to impaired maturation of the malignant clone, and thus MDS and many AML subtypes form a biological continuum rather than representing two distinct diseases. Recent data suggest that, in addition to previously described translocations, NPM1 mutations and KMT2A rearrangements are also AML-defining genetic alterations that lead to rapid disease progression, even if they present initially with less than 20% blasts. While some adult patients <20% blasts can be treated effectively with intensive AML-type chemotherapy, in the future, treatment of individual patients in this MDS/AML group will likely be dictated by genetic, biological, and patient-related factors rather than an arbitrary blast percentage.

Patients with MDS often suffer from anemia, and less often thrombocytopenia, and thus are a frequently transfused population. Red blood cell (RBC) transfusion may be used to improve functional capacity and quality of life in this population, while platelet transfusion is typically used to decrease bleeding risk. Despite the frequency of transfusion in patients with MDS, there are few well-defined guidelines for RBC and platelet transfusion support in this patient population. Transfusion is not without risk–patients with MDS who are frequently transfused may develop alloantibodies to RBC antigens, which can lead to hemolytic transfusion reactions and delays in obtaining compatible RBCs. Regular communication between clinicians and blood bank physicians is crucial to ensure that patients with MDS receive the most appropriate blood products.

The diagnosis of myelodysplastic syndromes/neoplasms (MDS) has evolved over the years with the incorporation of genetic abnormalities to establish a diagnosis, their impact on risk stratification, prognostication, and therapeutic options. Hematopathologists are the cornerstone to establish an accurate diagnosis and ensure patients receive the best available treatment option. Hematopathologists and clinicians must work closely together to establish the best disease subclassification, by combining pathologic findings with the clinical presentation. This will ensure patients receive the best therapeutic approach by better understanding the disease entity. In this review, we discuss how we approach a bone marrow biopsy report in the management of MDS.

CLINICS IN LABORATORY MEDICINE

SERIES OF RELATED INTEREST

Advances in Molecular Pathology
Available at: https://www.journals.elsevier.com/advances-in-molecular-pathology

---

THE CLINICS ARE NOW AVAILABLE ONLINE!
Access your subscription at:
www.theclinics.com

Preface

Advances in Myelodysplastic Syndromes

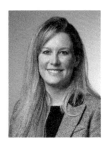

Alexa J. Siddon, MD
Editor

The practice of laboratory medicine is becoming increasingly specialized to accurately diagnose and ultimately care for patients, particularly in the era of personalized medicine. Myelodysplastic syndromes/neoplasms (MDS) have been a recognized group of clonal myeloid diseases for decades, with a continually evolving understanding of their pathogenesis. MDS was originally defined by morphology and the number of blasts in peripheral blood and marrow. Later, the incorporation of cytogenetics and fluorescence in situ hybridization testing further helped to refine subclassification. More recently, the routine evaluation of molecular alterations has been incorporated into the workup of cytopenic patients and has provided additional insight into the diagnosis, prognosis, and even therapy of patients ultimately diagnosed with MDS. In the past several years, the increased use of high-throughput molecular techniques, such as massively parallel sequencing (also known as next-generation sequencing), has allowed for the evaluation of numerous genes at once. This has led to an immense increase in our understanding of the molecular underpinnings that drive the course of disease. In 2022, the pathology/laboratory medicine and hematology communities received the newest updates to the guidelines for MDS, from both the fifth edition of the World Health Organization Classification of Haematolymphoid Tumors and the International Consensus Classification. Classifications continue to be based more heavily on molecular findings, including new diagnostic categories based on mutations in *SF3B1* and *TP53*. Molecular alterations are being used in conjunction with blast count to blur even the lines between MDS and Acute Myeloid Leukemia.

The evaluation and treatment of patients with MDS have become a truly multidisciplinary approach, which is reflected in this issue of *Clinics in Laboratory Medicine*. The authors of these articles are experts who take a deep dive into important aspects of MDS and highlight the specialization of their skills in diagnosis and treatment. It takes

Clin Lab Med 43 (2023) xiii–xiv
https://doi.org/10.1016/j.cll.2023.08.015
0272-2712/23/© 2023 Published by Elsevier Inc.

an array of primary care physicians, hematologists, hematopathologists, transfusion medicine specialists, molecular pathologists, and laboratory professionals to identify, diagnose, stratify, and effectively care for patients with MDS.

Alexa J. Siddon, MD
Department of Laboratory Medicine
& Pathology, Yale School of Medicine
New Haven, CT 06520, USA

E-mail address:
alexa.siddon@yale.edu

Flow Cytometric Assessment of Myelodysplastic Syndromes/Neoplasms

Xueyan Chen, MD, PhD[a,b], Ulrika Johansson, PhD[c],
Sindhu Cherian, MD[b,*]

KEYWORDS

- Myelodysplastic syndromes/neoplasms • MDS • Flow cytometry
- Immunophenotyping • Myeloid maturation

KEY POINTS

- Multiparametric flow cytometry (MFC) is a valuable tool that can assist in the diagnosis and characterization of myelodysplastic syndromes/neoplasms (MDS).
- MFC for identification of MDS relies on identifying immunophenotypic abnormalities that distinguish dysplastic populations from normal hematopoiesis on the basis of deviation of antigen expression from normal patterns seen during maturation and differentiation.
- Sensitivity of MFC for evaluating MDS is increased with incorporation of multiple informative parameters assessing several populations, including progenitor, maturing granulocytic, monocytic, and erythroid populations.
- Accurate assessment of specimens for MDS by MFC is improved with experience and requires a thorough understanding of the spectrum of immunophenotypic changes that accompany reactive processes.
- Advancements in standardization of all elements of testing from specimen processing to data analysis will make widespread use of MFC in MDS more feasible.

INTRODUCTION

During the process of hematopoiesis, hematopoietic stem cells (HSCs) undergo hierarchical differentiation and maturation to develop into mature effector cells through a tightly regulated process dictated by the interaction of underlying genetic and environmental factors. Hematopoietic cells of different lineages and maturation stages have

[a] Translational Science and Therapeutics Division, Fred Hutch Cancer Center, Seattle, WA, USA;
[b] Department of Laboratory Medicine and Pathology, University of Washington, 825 Eastlake Avenue East, Seattle, WA 98109, USA; [c] SI-HMDS, Haematology, UHBW NHS Foundation Trust, Bristol Royal Infirmary, Upper Maudlin Street, Bristol, BS2 8HW, UK
* Corresponding author. Hematopathology, G-7800, 825 Eastlake Avenue East, Seattle, WA 98109.
E-mail address: cherians@uw.edu

Clin Lab Med 43 (2023) 521–547
https://doi.org/10.1016/j.cll.2023.06.006
0272-2712/23/Crown Copyright © 2023 Published by Elsevier Inc. All rights reserved.

labmed.theclinics.com

characteristic morphologic and functional features. Differentiation and maturation are similarly associated with conserved and specific patterns of antigen expression, which can be interrogated by multiparametric flow cytometry (MFC). In hematopoietic neoplasms, such as myelodysplastic syndromes/neoplasms (MDS), in the same way that dysplasia is accompanied by abnormal morphology, hematopoietic cells can show altered patterns of antigen expression that deviate from that associated with normal hematopoiesis. The diagnosis and classification of MDS requires an integration of clinical, morphologic, and genetic data; immunophenotyping by MFC using a combination of reagents to assess antigenic shifts associated with normal and abnormal myeloid, monocytic, and erythroid maturation can assist in the work up for MDS. The value of MFC in the diagnosis of MDS has been demonstrated in numerous studies over the last 3 decades; however, challenges related to standardization have limited the widespread use of this methodology. Although the lack of well-established criteria beyond Ogata score[1,2] has limited the application of MFC in the diagnosis of MDS, there are ongoing efforts to standardize and harmonize methodologies and reagents, aiming to facilitate incorporation of this valuable tool in daily practice.

NORMAL MYELOID AND ERYTHROID MATURATION
Panel for Immunophenotyping

Antigen expression patterns seen during normal myeloid and erythroid maturation are highly reproducible and such normal patterns provide a baseline to distinguish abnormal cells with immunophenotypic aberrancies using MFC.[3–7] A desirable antibody panel would facilitate evaluation of precursor compartments as well as maturation of granulocytic, monocytic, and erythroid cells. The antibody panels currently used in our laboratories to evaluate myeloid neoplasms are listed in **Table 1**. Panel A includes antigens denoting immaturity to identify progenitors; antigens that are expressed at varying levels as progenitors differentiate into maturing granulocytic, monocytic, and erythroid forms; antigens for specific identification of other populations such as basophils, eosinophils, and plasmacytoid dendritic cells (PDCs); and lymphoid antigens to evaluate aberrant cross-lineage antigen expression on progenitors and to exclude a lymphoproliferative disorder. Detailed immunophenotypic analysis of progenitors and maturing populations would demonstrate characteristic antigen expression patterns during normal hematopoiesis and allow recognition of abnormal patterns associated with myeloid neoplasms. A variety of approaches have been employed for characterizing myelomonocytic maturation and recently a 1-tube 10-antibody panel (CD10, CD11b, CD13, CD14, CD16, CD33, CD34, CD45, CD56, and CD64) has been described in the literature and validated to evaluate granulocytic and monocytic maturation as a sensitive and specific tool for the diagnosis of MDS[8] (see **Table 1**). Panel B highlights antigens important for assessment of erythroid maturation. Erythroid evaluation often begins by using CD45, CD71, and CD117 to identify erythroid precursors with additional antigens incorporated to define erythroid aberrancies.[9–11]

POPULATION IDENTIFICATION

CD45 versus side scatter (SSC) gating is commonly used as an initial strategy for hematopoietic cell identification,[6,12] allowing for discrimination of myeloid blasts, B lymphoid precursors (hematogones), mature lymphocytes, monocytes, and maturing granulocytes (**Fig. 1**). Progenitor populations typically express lower CD45 compared with mature cells and have intermediate SSC,[3] allowing enrichment of progenitors by

Table 1
Antibody panels for the evaluation of myeloid neoplasms

Panel A

Laser	Violet					Blue					Red		
Fluorochromes	PB/V450/BV421	BV510	BV605	BV711	BV786	A488	FITC	PE	PE-Cy5	PE-Cy7	APC	APC-A700	APC-H7
Myeloid 1	HLA-DR	CD38	CD19	CD33			CD15	CD117		CD13	CD34	CD71	CD45
Myeloid 2	HLA-DR	CD38	CD4		CD14		CD64	CD123		CD13	CD34	CD16	CD45
Myeloid 3	HLA-DR	CD38	CD5			CD56		CD7		CD33	CD34		CD45
B cell	CD20	CD38	CD5	CD200	CD3+CD56		Kappa	Lambda		CD19	CD10		CD45
T cell	CD8	CD38	CD5	CD4	CD7		CD2	CD5	CD56	CD3	CD34	CD30	CD45

Panel B

Laser	Violet		Blue				Red	
Fluorochromes	V500-C	BV421	FITC	PE	PerCP-Cy5.5	PE-Cy7	APC	APC-H7
Erythroid	CD45	HLA-DR	CD36	CD105	CD34	CD117	CD33	CD71

APC, allophycocyanin; BV, brilliant violet; FITC, fluorescein isothiocyanate; PB, pacific blue; PE, phycoerytherin; PE-Cy5, PE-Cyanine-5; PerCp-Cy5.5, Peridinin chlorophyll protein-Cyanine 5.5; PE-Cy7, PE-cyanine-7.

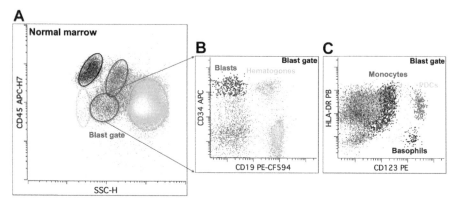

Fig. 1. Population identification by flow cytometry. (*A*) Using flow cytometry for population identification, CD45 versus SSC is a common initial gating strategy and provides a useful starting point to distinguish 5 major hematopoietic cell populations: mature lymphocytes (blue), monocytes (pink), maturing granulocytes (green), myeloid blasts (red), and B-cell precursors (hematogones; aqua). Cells in "blast gate" defined by dim CD45 and SSC contain more than just CD34-positive blasts; additional markers are required to differentiate these populations from normal progenitors. (*B*) Hematogones (aqua) and myeloid blasts (highlighted in red) can be separated by CD34 versus CD19. (*C*) Basophils (highlighted in purple), PDCs (highlighted in orange), and monocytes (highlighted in pink) can be separated by HLA-DR versus CD123.

creating a blast region on a plot of CD45 versus SSC. However, it is important to note that several other non-progenitor populations may reside in "blast gate" due to expression of similar levels of CD45 and SSC. Such populations may include basophils, PDCs, hypogranular neutrophils, immature monocytes, and plasma cells (see **Fig. 1**). Therefore, inclusion of additional antibodies in the panel to further dissect the populations falling within the "blast gate" is required to achieve a relatively pure progenitor population for further characterization.

Granulocytic Maturation

Hematopoiesis starts with a HSC in the bone marrow, which undergoes either self-renewal or multiple stages of differentiation, including multipotent progenitors, lineage committed progenitors with decreasing potential, and common myeloid or lymphoid progenitors. These progress into mature red blood cells, leukocytes, and platelets.[13] The HSC is characterized by a high level of CD34 expression, low to absent CD38 expression, a slightly higher level of CD45, and lower levels of CD13, CD33, CD71, CD117, CD123, and HLA-DR than the committed myeloid progenitors. HSCs lack high level expression of lineage-specific markers.[14,15] Through the transition from stem cells to common myeloid progenitors, CD38 expression increases while CD34 and CD45 expression gradually decreases, at which point progenitor cells start to express markers indicating lineage commitment.

Similar to the changes in morphology noted during normal granulocytic maturation, myeloid progenitors and maturing myelomonocytic cells demonstrate a conserved and coordinated pattern of antigen expression with progressive gains and losses of antigens in a continuous manner.[16] Changes in intensity of various antigens occur throughout all stages of development from stem cell to granulocytes. As early progenitors progress to promyelocytes, CD34-positive progenitors gradually acquire higher levels of CD13, CD33, CD38, and CD117 accompanied by decreased CD34, CD45,

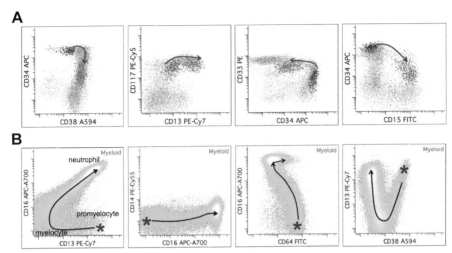

Fig. 2. Normal granulocytic maturation in bone marrow. (*A*) From stem cell to promyelocyte. The earliest progenitors (stem cell, highlighted in purple) express bright CD34, dim CD13, dim CD33, and dim CD38 without CD15. With differentiation, the progenitors gradually lose CD34 while acquiring CD15 and higher levels of CD13, CD33, and CD38, and reach promyelocyte stage (highlighted in orange). (*B*) From promyelocyte to neutrophil. The black line follows the changes in intensity of antigen expression as promyelocytes (star) develop to neutrophils (tip of *arrow*). With maturation, promyelocytes gradually lose CD13 till they reach the myelocyte stage, then re-acquire CD13 in conjunction with CD16 and reach neutrophil stage. CD38 and CD64 levels gradually decrease during this process.

and HLA-DR, and gain of CD15 and CD64 (**Fig. 2**A). During the transition from the promyelocyte to neutrophil stage, promyelocytes with high levels of CD13, CD33, and CD64 gradually decrease intensity of these antigens. CD13 expression is lost as cells reach the myelocyte stage. Subsequent maturation is characterized by simultaneous re-acquisition of CD13 in conjunction with CD16, which both reach high levels in mature neutrophils (**Fig. 2**B). Although CD64 intensity generally decreases with maturation from the promyelocyte to the neutrophil stage, upregulation of CD64 by cytokines has been described on mature neutrophils in inflammatory and infectious responses.[17]

Monocytic Maturation

As progenitors commit to the monocytic lineage, CD34 and CD117 decrease in intensity and cells begin to express high levels of CD11b, CD33, CD64, and HLA-DR;[3,7,16] the levels of CD33 and CD64 are higher on monocytic lineage cells than are seen on promyelocytes.[18] Immature monocytes (monoblasts and promonocytes) represent a low percentage of total nucleated cells in a normal bone marrow, expressing intermediate CD15 with low to absent CD13 and CD14, and typically lacking CD34 and CD117. The lack of CD14 is considered as a feature of immature monocytes that can provide evidence of immaturity, in particular, in cases where the morphologic distinction between immature monocytes and reactive mature monocytes is challenging. However, given that different clones of anti-CD14 antibody recognize different epitopes that appear at different maturation stage of monocytes, the detection of CD14 expression is significantly affected by the choice of the antibody clone.[19] Furthermore, the absence of CD14 on a proportion or even the majority of monocytes may indicate the presence of glycosylphosphatidylinositol (GPI)-deficient monocytes, which can be seen in conditions such as aplastic anemia, MDS, or paroxysmal nocturnal hemoglobinuria (PNH).[20,21] This is particularly important to recognize when the absence of CD14 is observed on otherwise mature monocytes. With maturation, monocytes express higher levels of CD13, CD14, CD45, and both CD300e and CD312. Mature monocytes are composed of several subsets including classical (CD14[hi]/CD300e[hi]/CD16-), intermediate (CD14[hi]/CD300e[hi]/CD16+), and non-classical (CD14[lo]/CD300e[hi]/CD16+) monocytes that have different functional capacity and may vary in proportion in different clinical settings.[22-24]

ERYTHROID MATURATION

As HSCs progress to early erythroid progenitors, CD33 expression is lost and intensity of CD34, CD45, and HLA-DR decreases, whereas expression of CD71, CD117, CD105, and CD36 increases as does glycophorin A (CD235a). At this point, the SSC of the cells also increases. With further maturation, CD117 begins to decrease and is eventually lost, and CD38, CD45, and CD105 decrease, accompanied by a sharp drop is SSC. With progression to the reticulocyte stage, CD105 expression is fully lost, and this is eventually followed by a loss of both CD71 and CD36 as the mature anucleated red blood cell stage is reached (**Fig. 3**).[9-11,25-32] Notably, glycophorin A is retained through the mature red blood cell stage. Use of anti-glycophorin A antibody may result in red cell

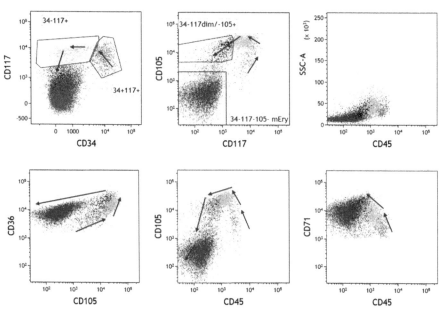

Fig. 3. Normal erythroid maturation in bone marrow. The plots demonstrate erythroid maturation patterns in normal bone marrow. CD34-positive early erythroid progenitors (red) are CD117+, CD71 dim+, CD36 dim+ and CD105-/dim+. As they mature, CD36, CD71, CD105, and SSC increase, whereas CD45 expression decreases and the CD34 expression is lost, resulting in a CD34-/CD117+/CD71+/CD36+/++/CD105++/CD45 dim + stage (green). This is followed by continued decrease in CD117 and CD45 and decreased CD105, whereas the CD71 expression peaks (blue). CD117 is then lost, followed by loss of CD45, and CD105 decreases until finally only CD36 and CD71 remain (maroon/brown). The final step, loss of CD71 and CD36, is not depicted in this figure.

aggregation, as is well described for peripheral blood red cell PNH analysis.[33] Similar issues may be seen in bone marrow analysis and if glycophorin A is used to map erythroid maturation patterns in bone marrow samples, a Lyse-Wash-Label-Wash type protocol is required to achieve consistent results.[34] It should be noted that most processing methods result in a selective loss of particularly the maturing erythroid cells so that proportionally, a differential quantification of cell lineages by MFC will nearly always produce artificially low erythroid cell count compared with the cytomorphology differential count.[35] That said, studying the antigen expression patterns and light scatter properties of the maturing erythroid cell in bone marrow is very informative for MDS analysis.

IMMUNOPHENOTYPIC ABNORMALITIES ASSOCIATED WITH MYELODYSPLASTIC SYNDROMES/NEOPLASMS

MDS are a heterogeneous group of clonal stem cell disorders characterized by peripheral cytopenias, dysplasia, and increased risk of progression to acute myeloid leukemia (AML).[36] Classification of MDS using the 5th edition World Health Organization (WHO-HAEM5) and International Consensus Classification (ICC) classification systems is based on an integration of clinical, morphologic, and genetic criteria; MFC can assist in diagnosis, classification, prognosis, and disease monitoring. The rationale of application of MFC in the diagnosis of MDS relies on the ability of MFC to distinguish immunophenotypically abnormal myeloid blasts and aberrant maturation patterns from normal counterparts. Specific recommendations for integrating MFC into the diagnostic work up for MDS have been proposed by the International/European LeukemiaNet Working Group for Flow Cytometry in MDS (ELN/iMDS Flow) and have been reviewed recently with the recommendations to evaluate myeloid blasts, granulocytic and monocytic maturation, and erythropoiesis using a comprehensive panel.[31,34,37,38]

ABNORMALITIES ON MYELOID PROGENITORS

In MDS, an increase in myeloid progenitors is a common finding with prognostic significance.[31,38–40] WHO-HAEM5 and ICC indicate thresholds for blast percentage that is associated with different MDS subtypes and with prognosis and likelihood of progression to AML. Assessment of blast percentage by MFC may be hampered by factors including hemodilution and partial lysis of erythroid precursors during specimen processing.[41,42] Although the former can lead to underrepresentation of the blast percentage, the latter can lead to overestimation of the blast percentage compared with morphology, in particular, in cases with relative erythroid hyperplasia in the background. Despite these factors, blast quantification by MFC provides an objective, reliable diagnostic and prognostic measurement in MDS by a recent study.[43] A prospective multicenter study of the ELN/iMDS Flow revealed that when controlling for factors including hemodilution and specimen processing, the presence of greater than 3% myeloid progenitors (defined as CD34+ progenitors lacking CD19) in diagnostic (treatment naïve) specimens was significantly associated with MDS; therefore, a cut-off of 3% blasts was suggested by this group.[38] It is critical to note that preanalytic factors including specimen age and degree of hemodilution, as well as methodologic differences in specimen processing can significantly impact percentages; therefore, care should be taken when establishing such a threshold. Further, as noted below, blast percentage can increase with marrow recovery post induction therapy or with administration of growth factors, particularly in younger individuals; therefore, such numeric criteria are not reliable in these settings.

Aberrant immunophenotypic features in myeloid progenitors in MDS generally fall into 1 of the 4 categories[3]: (1) abnormal levels of antigen expression (increased or decreased intensity, or complete loss); (2) asynchronous expression of immature and differentiation antigens, for example, co-expression of antigens associated with maturation, such as CD15 or CD64, on progenitors expressing high levels of CD34; (3) homogenous expression of antigens normally expressed at varying levels during maturation; (4) expression of antigens associated with other lineages (cross-lineage antigen expression), such as CD2, CD4, CD5, CD7, CD19, and/or CD56.[44–46] **Fig. 4** shows an abnormal blast population from a patient with MDS with abnormal expression of multiple antigens. Data from the aforementioned prospective multicenter study identified a total of 17 immunophenotypic markers that were independently related to MDS, and cases with greater than or equal to 3 of these aberrancies showed 80% concordance with cytomorphology, emphasizing the clinical utility of MFC in the diagnosis of MDS.[38] Abnormal expression of CD117, CD45, CD34, CD7, CD13, CD33, and CD5 were the most frequent aberrancies in both low-risk and high-risk MDS. Compared with reactive alterations that are relatively mild and often only involve a single antigen, immunophenotypic abnormalities associated with MDS frequently involve multiple antigens and the degree of deviation from normal patterns is more prominent.

Myeloid neoplasms derive from malignant stem cells that arise due to underlying genetic and epigenetic alterations in HSCs.[47–52] In MDS, the CD34++/CD38 dim to absent stem cell subset (as a proportion of all CD34+ progenitors) may be relatively increased. This is thought by some to reflect reduced heterogeneity in the progenitor compartment, a finding that also leads to the observation of decreased normal B-cell precursors (hematogones) in MDS.[53] Normal HSCs are characterized by CD34++, CD38-, CD45RA-, and CD90+.[54] In addition to being proportionally increased, stem cells may harbor significant immunophenotypic abnormalities in MDS. **Fig. 5A** highlights a normal HSC population that has bright CD34, dim CD38, higher CD45, lower

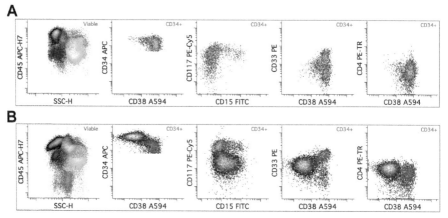

Fig. 4. Immunophenotypic abnormalities on myeloid blasts in MDS. (*A*) Normal bone marrow. The CD34+ blasts (red) show a normal expression pattern of CD4, CD15, CD33 CD34, CD38, and CD117. (*B*) Bone marrow from a patient with MDS. The CD34+ myeloid blasts represent 2.4% of the white cells and include an aberrant subset (purple) comprising 1.6% of the white blood cells. The aberrant blasts (purple) show abnormal expression of CD34 (increased, uniform), CD38 (decreased), CD15 (dim), CD33 (decreased, uniform), and CD4 (mildly increased, uniform). A relatively normal CD34+ myeloid progenitor population (red) is also present in the background.

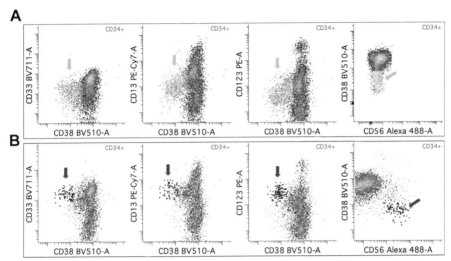

Fig. 5. Immunophenotypic abnormalities on stem cells in MDS. All plots show CD34-positive cells. (*A*) CD34-positive blasts from a normal bone marrow. The blasts include a subset of stem cells (aqua) with lower CD33, lower CD38, lower CD13, and lower CD123 compared to the rest of the blasts (*red*). (*B*) CD34-positive blasts from the bone marrow of a patient with MDS. The stem cell subset (highlighted in purple) shows aberrant expression of CD33 (mildly increased), CD13 (mildly increased), CD123 (increased), and CD56. The rest of the blasts (*red*) show a normal antigen expression pattern.

CD117, lower CD13, and lower CD123 than rest of the myeloid progenitors. In contrast, **Fig. 5**B shows an example of abnormal stem cells from a patient with MDS. Aberrant expression of several differentiation and T lineage antigens may be seen in MDS with aberrant expression of CLL-1, CD44, CD47, and CD123 reported in high-grade MDS.[49,55,56]

ABNORMALITIES ON MATURING GRANULOCYTIC CELLS

Immunophenotypic aberrancies on maturing granulocytic cells are frequently identified in MDS. Hypogranularity of neutrophils is one of the major dysplastic features recognized by cytomorphology and can be detected by MFC as a decrease in neutrophil SSC or by a decrease in the ratio of SSC between maturing granulocytic cells and mature lymphocytes.[1,2,57,58] Eosinophils, which have high SSC and lack CD16, must be excluded from granulocyte gating to ensure accurate SSC analysis of neutrophils. Decreased expression of CD45,[8,39] decreased expression or absence of CD10,[8,59,60] decreased expression or absence of CD33,[39,45,61,62] increased expression of CD14 and CD64,[8,39,62,63] and cross-lineage expression of lymphoid markers (CD5, CD7, CD19, and CD56)[8,45,61] on maturing granulocytic cells have also been reported in MDS. Asynchronous expression of progenitor -related antigens, such as CD34 and CD117, on maturing granulocytic cells has been reported in MDS.[45,61,64] These individual aberrancies are not specific and may be seen in other reactive conditions. Therefore, evaluating a combination of markers and assessing maturation patterns is necessary to distinguish reactive aberrancies from MDS associated abnormalities. Notably, abnormal granulocytic maturation patterns, including dyssynchronous expression of CD13/CD16 and CD13/CD11b, occur more frequently in MDS than in hospitalized control patients.[38] **Fig. 6** demonstrates an abnormal granulocytic

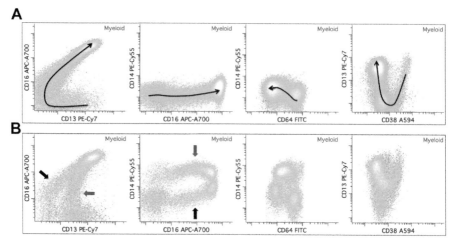

Fig. 6. Abnormal granulocytic maturation in MDS. All plots show maturing granulocytic cells. (*A*) Normal bone marrow. The black line follows the changes in intensity of antigen expression during granulocytic maturation. (*B*) Bone marrow from an MDS patient with monosomy 7. The maturing granulocytic cells show 2 lines of maturation. In addition to a normal subset (highlighted by the *black arrow*), an additional abnormal line of granulocytic maturation (highlighted by the *red arrow*) is noted with increased CD13 and CD14 expression.

maturation pattern in MDS. Of note, eosinophilia in bone marrow may be present in some MDS cases. Aberrant immunophenotypic features of eosinophils in MDS have not been defined. It has been recommended by the ELN/iMDS Flow that evaluation of granulocytes should include quantification, granulocyte SSC, expression of CD33 and CD13/CD16 pattern, all of which were independently associated with a diagnosis of MDS.[38]

Abnormalities on Monocytic Cells

In MDS, immunophenotypic alterations on monocytic cells occur less frequently than those seen in the progenitor compartment and on maturing granulocytic cells. In some subtypes of MDS or MDS/myeloproliferative neoplasm overlap syndromes (MDS/MPN) with dysplastic and proliferative features such as chronic myelomonocytic leukemia (CMML), monocytic forms may be proportionally increased and/or show left shifted maturation.[65,66] The monocyte aberrations frequently described include an increase or decrease in the percentage of monocytes, decreased SSC (20%–30% of MDS cases),[39] abnormal intensities of antigens normally expressed on monocytic cells including CD13, CD14, CD15, CD33, CD45, CD64, and HLA-DR,[34,38,39,64,67,68] and decreased proportion of CD14 and/or CD300e + mature monocytes.[39] Monocytic cells may have aberrant expression of lymphoid antigens, such as CD5, CD7, CD19, and CD56 with aberrant CD56 being most commonly reported.[39,64,67] Based on currently available data, evaluation of monocytic cells in MDS should include quantification, expression of CD13 and CD56, and expression pattern of HLA-DR/CD11b, which have been shown to be associated with a diagnosis of MDS or MDS/MPN.[38]

CMML and other MDS/MPN with both dysplastic and proliferative features typically associated with a relative and absolute monocytosis may be accompanied by characteristic changes in monocytic subsets in the peripheral blood. Notably, in contrast to reactive monocytic proliferations, CMML has a higher proportion of classical monocytes (CD14^{hi}/CD16–) (**Fig. 7**), with some studies suggesting that a classical monocyte

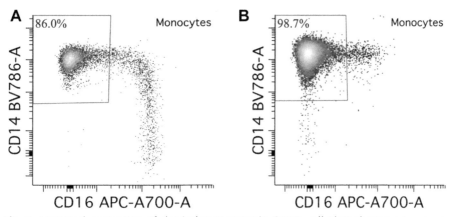

Fig. 7. Increased proportion of classical monocytes in CMML. All plots show monocytes in the peripheral blood. Classical monocytes are highlighted in orange. (*A*). Monocytes from a patient with reactive monocytosis. (*B*) Monocytes from a patient with CMML. The proportion of classical monocytes (monocytes expressing bright CD14 without CD16) accounts for greater than or equal to 94% of monocytes.

proportion of greater than or equal to 94% in the peripheral blood is highly specific for CMML.[69–72] Investigators have demonstrated the utility of this approach in the marrow; however, work conducted by the ELN/iMDS Flow suggests that the high sensitivity and specificity of the peripheral blood monocyte partitioning assay are not maintained when evaluating bone marrow samples.[72]

Abnormalities on Erythroid Precursors

The first described and probably best documented MDS-related abnormalities in the erythroid compartment are changes in CD71 expression on the CD34-negative/CD117-negative/CD45 dim to negative maturing erythroid cells.[11,73–76] The bright and reasonably homogeneous CD71 expression on erythroid cells that is seen in normal marrows or non-clonal cytopenias is often replaced by a "waterfall" or "comet tail" type of heterogeneous expression pattern in MDS. This can be measured as an increased coefficient of variation (CV) and reduced median fluorescent intensity (MdFI). Similarly, CD36 expression on the maturing erythroid cells in MDS may be heterogeneous and reduced compared with that seen in normal marrow. A multicenter study that specifically evaluated erythroid abnormalities in MDS versus normal or non-clonal cytopenia found a higher statistical difference between normal/non-clonal cytopenias and MDS when comparing the values for CD36 CV rather than CD36 MdFI, suggesting that the heterogeneity of this protein expression across the maturing erythroid cells is a stronger indicator of dyserythropoiesis than its expression intensity.[76] Examples of abnormal erythroid maturation are shown in **Fig. 8**.

The erythroid compartment is generally less well studied compared with the myeloid lineages. And so, to date no other protein expression pattern has consistently been shown to differ between MDS and normal bone marrows. However, the light scatter properties of the erythroid compartment have been demonstrated to be altered in MDS: The CD34-negative/CD117-negative/CD45 dim to negative maturing erythroid cells in MDS frequently have increased SSC compared with normal and non-clonal cytopenias.[77] This may be found across low-grade MDS entities and is described as a feature of MDS with SF3B1 mutation.[78] A caveat here is megaloblastic anemia, where an increased SSC could be present. In such circumstances, the overall antigen

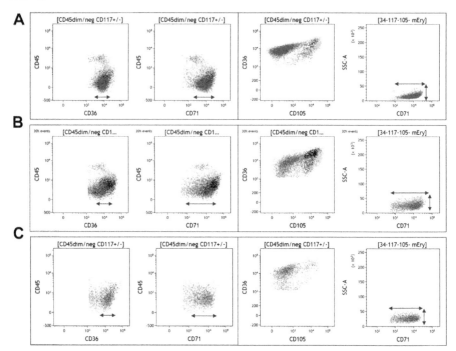

Fig. 8. Abnormal erythroid maturation in MDS. All plots show erythroid cells in bone marrow. (*A*) Normal erythroid maturation. Maturing erythroid cells that have reached the CD34-/CD117-/CD105-stage (maroon) have a reasonably homogeneous CD36 expression whereas more heterogeneous CD71 expression. The SSC is low. (*B*) MDS with mutated *SF3B1*. The maturing erythroid forms (maroon) show an increased CV for CD71 and CD36, and increased SSC. (*C*) MDS, low grade. Again, compared with the normal example, the maturing erythroid cells show an increased CV for CD71 and CD36, and increased SSC.

maturation profile is expected to be within normal limits, though a left-shifted phenotype may be present. The overall relative proportion of erythroid cells, and of erythroid progenitors within the erythroid compartment, may be increased, reflecting erythroid hyperplasia. An increase or a decrease in the relative proportion of immature (CD117+ or CD105+) erythroid precursors of the total erythroid compartment, and/or of the total progenitor cell compartment, may also be present in MDS. This finding is often accompanied by the presence of further typical MDS-associated abnormalities throughout the erythroid and other lineages, and the demonstration of multiple abnormalities would increase specificity. It should be mentioned here that erythroid hyperplasia together with a prominent, and phenotypically abnormal erythroblast population, raises possibility of acute erythroid leukemia as does presence of a prominent, phenotypically abnormal erythroblast population in the absence of general erythroid hyperplasia.[29]

IMMUNOPHENOTYPIC ABNORMALITIES ASSOCIATED WITH GENETIC ABERRATIONS

In AML, a strong correlation has been established between specific immunophenotypic profiles and underlying genetic abnormalities, including t(15;17),[79–83] t(8;21),[84–86] *FLT3* internal tandem duplication,[87,88] and *NPM1* mutation.[79,80,82,89] Because of the heterogeneity of MDS and wide genetic landscape, associations between genetic aberration and distinct immunophenotypic profiles are not well established in majority of entities within MDS. We review below available data relating to phenotype-genotype correlations in MDS.

Abnormalities Associated with Monosomy 7

Chromosome 7 abnormalities are recurrent cytogenetic aberrations frequently detected in MDS.[36] Monosomy 7 is designated as a poor risk cytogenetic aberration and deletion 7q in the intermediate risk group by revised International Prognostic Scoring System (R-IPSS).[90] A comprehensive MFC analysis of myeloid neoplasms harboring chromosome 7 abnormalities recognized increased CD14 on maturing granulocytic cells as the most frequent aberrations associated with monosomy 7 but not deletion 7q (92.9% vs 8.2%).[63] Patients may have increased CD14 at all stages of granulocytic maturation, or have 2 lines of granulocytic maturation, one with normal CD14, and one with increased intensity of CD14 expression (**Fig. 6**B). CD64 retention was also more frequently observed in monosomy 7 than in deletion 7q. Besides CD14 and CD64 aberrations, a list of other abnormalities was also identified in myeloid blasts and maturing myelomonocytic cells, although there was no significance difference in frequencies of these abnormalities between monosomy 7 and deletion 7q. Recognition of immunophenotypic features can assist in evaluation of this disease by MFC, in particular, in patients with low blast count or minimal immunophenotypic alterations on myeloid blasts. The underlying mechanism of the reproducible abnormalities associated with monosomy 7 is yet to be explored.

Abnormalities Associated with SF3B1

MDS with mutated *SF3B1* is recognized as a distinct entity by WHO-HAEM5[91] and ICC classification.[92] Immunophenotypic features associated with MDS with mutations *SF3B1* have been described, including increased percentage of erythroid precursors and mast cells, abnormal expression of CD71 (higher CV and lower MdFI) (**Fig. 8**B), increased SSC on erythroid and myeloid progenitors, decreased CD11b expression on neutrophils, and decreased expression of CD11b, CD36, and CD64 on monocytes.[78] *SF3B1* K700 E mutation is associated with significantly lower CD11b on monocytes and neutrophils, higher percentage of masts cells, and lower CD36 on monocytes compared with other *SF3B1* mutations. Given the specific genotype-phenotype association, *SF3B1* mutation subtype may have impact on disease pathogenesis and treatment response.

Abnormalities Associated with del(5q)

MDS with isolated del(5q) remains as a distinct MDS subtype in WHO-HAEM5[91] and ICC classification with characteristic cytomorphologic features.[92] A 5-parameter scoring system including CD45-MdFI-ratio (lymphocytes vs myeloid precursors; $\leq$ 7.0, 10 points), percentage of myeloid precursors (>2.0%, 3 points), granulocytes versus lymphocytes SSC ratio (<6.0, 2 points), CD71 expression on granulocytes ($\leq$20%, 1.5 points), and sex (female, 1.5 points) was validated in MDS with del(5q).[93] A score of 15.0 or more was strongly associated with the presence of del(5q) and a score less than 10 never identified in del(5q) MDS. The 5-parameter score was tested in monitoring treatment response to lenalidomide-based therapy in a subset of patients with del(5q) MDS. The score remained high (mean = 16.5) in patients not achieving complete cytogenetic response (cCR), but was decreased (mean score = 13.0) in all patients achieving cCR. The scoring system may be incorporated into MDS diagnostics as a complimentary, fast tool to confirm the diagnosis.

SF3B1 mutations co-occur in 20% of MDS with del(5q).[94] In patients with MDS with both del(5q) and *SF3B1* mutation, some immunophenotypic features were reported to be more similar to del(5q) MDS, including erythroid precursor percentage and CD71 expression, CD38 and CD117 levels on progenitors, and percentage of lymphocytes, whereas CD11b, CD14, and CD36 levels on monocytes and CD11b level on neutrophils were more similar to those seen in MDS with *SF3B1* mutation.[78]

IMMUNOPHENOTYPIC ALTERATIONS IN REACTIVE/REGENERATIVE CONDITIONS

Immunophenotypic alterations can be observed in blasts and maturing granulocytic and monocytic cells in a variety of reactive conditions. It is critical to distinguish atypical antigen expression patterns associated with reactive conditions from abnormalities associated with myeloid neoplasms for accurate interpretation. In some cases, changes seen in reactive settings may overlap with that seen in association with MDS; therefore, immunophenotypic changes should be considered in the appropriate clinical and morphologic context. Examples of non-neoplastic immunophenotypic alterations that may be encountered on myelomonocytic populations are reviewed below.

Marrow Regeneration and granulocyte colony stimulating factor (G-CSF) Effect

Reactive immunophenotypic alterations have been described in marrow regeneration which may be seen post cytotoxic chemotherapy or in the setting of a toxic/autoimmune/infectious marrow insult either with or without G-CSF administration.[3,16,95,96] Regenerative bone marrow often demonstrates a marked myeloid left shift, expansion of late stage committed myeloid progenitor/early promyelocyte populations, relatively synchronous maturation of the progenitors manifested by homogeneous expression of antigens normally expressed at heterogeneous levels through maturation including CD33, CD34, CD38 and HLA-DR, and by heterogeneous CD56 expression on maturing granulocytic and monocytic cells.[16] In the setting of G-CSF administration, changes similar to that described above may be seen. In addition, other unique features have been reported and include an expansion of a myeloid blast population with decreased expression of CD33, CD38, and HLA-DR; dyssynchronous expression of CD13 and CD16 on maturing granulocytic cells; increased CD14 expression on maturing granulocytic cells[63]; and decreased SSC on maturing granulocytic cells[16,96] (**Fig. 9**). Knowledge of normal and reactive patterns of antigen expression in the setting of marrow regeneration and growth factor treatment is crucial to accurately discriminate neoplastic abnormalities from benign conditions, in particular, in light of the widespread use of G-CSF in neutropenic patients in current clinical practice.

Glycosylphosphatidylinositol-Deficient Granulocytes and Monocytes

Patients with PNH may have decreased to absent expression of GPI-linked proteins which can alter expression of antigens used to evaluate lineage and maturational stages of myelomonocytic cells. For instance, GPI-linked proteins CD16 and CD14 are commonly used to evaluate neutrophilic and monocytic maturation; however, in the setting of PNH, CD16 will be reduced on a subset of mature neutrophils and CD14 will show reduced expression on a subset of mature monocytes.[97] The presence of GPI-deficient granulocytes and monocytes in bone marrow makes use of CD16 and CD14 to evaluate maturation of granulocytic cells and monocytes challenging and changes typical antigenic patterns associated with normal maturation (**Fig. 10A**). It is important to recognize the pattern of PNH in the bone marrow to avoid

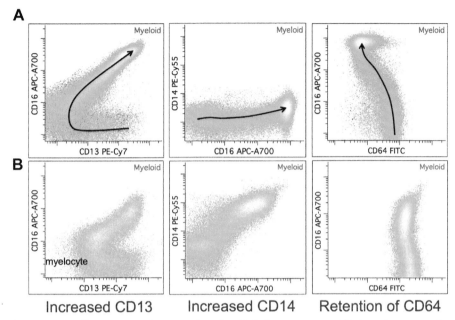

Increased CD13   Increased CD14   Retention of CD64

Fig. 9. G-CSF effect on maturing granulocytic cells in bone marrow. All plots show maturing granulocytic cells. (*A*) Normal bone marrow. The black line follows the changes in intensity of antigen expression during granulocytic maturation. (*B*) After G-CSF administration, the maturing granulocytic cells in bone marrow show increased CD13 expression forming a right angle like shape to the pattern rather than the characteristic smoothly curved pattern, and retention of CD64.

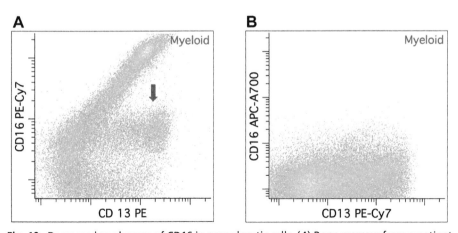

Fig. 10. Decreased or absence of CD16 in granulocytic cells. (*A*) Bone marrow from a patient with PNH. A subset of neutrophils show decreased expression of CD16 (red *arrow*), representing GPI-deficient neutrophils. (*B*) In an otherwise normal bone marrow from a patient with mild neutropenia, all maturing granulocytic cells in bone marrow show complete loss of CD16 expression. CD16 is expressed on NK cells at a normal level and on non-classical monocytes (data not shown).

mistaking this as MDS. If a pattern of antigen expression suggesting PNH is identified, peripheral blood testing is warranted to confirm the diagnosis and quantify the GPI-deficient clones following available guidelines.[97] It should be noted that small GPI-deficient clones may be present in a subset of patients with aplastic anemia and/or MDS.[20,21] As GPI-deficient populations seen in this setting are typically relatively small, the presence of these populations often does not significantly impact the overall myelomonocytic maturation pattern.

Occasionally, complete loss of CD16 expression on neutrophils but not on NK cells or monocytes may be detected in an otherwise healthy individual (**Fig. 10**B). The plausible causes of isolated loss of CD16 on neutrophils include absence or mutation in the FcRIII-1 gene encoding GPI-linked CD16 protein expressed on neutrophils, FcRIII-1 gene polymorphism, or defective post-translational modification of the protein product of this gene resulting in absence of CD16 epitopes required for antibody recognition.[98–100]

Effect of Targeted Therapy

Increased implementation of targeted immunotherapy in a variety of hematolymphoid neoplasms has substantially improved patients' outcomes. However, targeted immunotherapy can lead to immunophenotypic shifts on blasts and maturing granulocytic and monocytic populations, resulting in an altered pattern of antigen expression that deviates from normal. Daratumumab is a human monoclonal antibody against CD38 and has been widely used in the treatment of multiple myeloma.[101] Daratumumab may be persistently present on the cell surface of CD38-expressing cells for several months after treatment discontinuation.[102] Because of the overlap between the diagnostic CD38 antibody and daratumumab binding sites, the presence of daratumumab interferes with flow cytometric detection of CD38, resulting in apparent loss of CD38 in all CD38-expressing cells (**Fig. 11**). This can cause a particular challenge as CD38 is often used in conjunction with CD34 to identify normal and aberrant stem cell

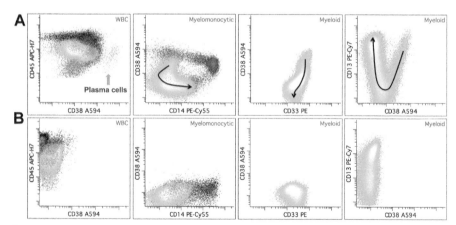

Fig. 11. Immunophenotypic alterations on maturing granulocytic cells and monocytes in bone marrow post targeted therapy. (*A*) In normal bone marrow, all populations express CD38; plasma cells (green *arrow*) have highest level of CD38. Maturing granulocytic cells and monocytes demonstrate a normal antigen expression pattern of CD38 versus other informative antigens. (*B*) Post daratumumab (anti-CD38) therapy, all populations in bone marrow lose CD38 expression, resulting in an antigenic pattern change in CD38 versus CD14, CD38 versus CD33, and CD13 versus CD38 plots.

populations which, as noted above, can be proportionally increased in MDS. In the current therapeutic environment, it is critically important to be aware of treatment history to recognize therapeutic effects on myeloid cells and distinguish such effects from aberrancies associated with myelodysplasia.

Regenerative Changes Associated with Trisomy 21

Down syndrome (DS) is characterized by constitutional trisomy 21 and has an increased risk of developing AML.[36] The progenitors and maturing myelomonocytic cells in patients with DS have a unique immunophenotype. Aberrant CD56 expression is present on myeloid progenitors, maturing granulocytes and monocytes in the majority of DS cases.[103–105] In DS patients with myeloid leukemia in complete remission post chemotherapy, granulocytes and monocytes show increased CD33 expression and aberrant expression of CD56, with overexpression of RUNX1.[104] Absence of HLA-DR may be seen in subset of blasts. Although CD56 expression on blasts is often regarded as an aberrant feature, CD56 expression on blasts and maturing myelomonocytic cells in DS is an inherent feature associated with regeneration and therefore should not be deemed as immunophenotypic evidence of either dysplasia, or measurable residual disease during disease monitoring.[106] **Fig. 12**A illustrates a post-treatment, pre-transplant remission marrow from a DS patient with AML, which show aberrant CD56 expression on myeloid blasts, monocytes, and granulocytes. The aberrancies present in the pre-transplant marrow are not observed in the post-transplant marrow with a normal karyotype (**Fig. 12**B).

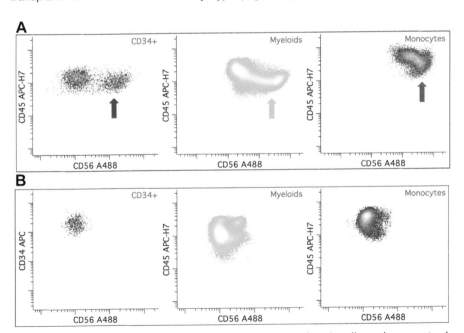

Fig. 12. CD56 expression on myeloid blasts, maturing granulocytic cells, and monocytes in Down syndrome. (*A*) Pre-transplant remission bone marrow from a patient with Down syndrome with a history of acute myeloid leukemia. CD56 is expressed on a subset of blasts (*red arrow*) and on a subset of maturing granulocytic cells (*green arrow*) and monocytes (*pink arrow*). (*B*) Day 28 post-transplant bone marrow. The CD56 expression seen in the pre-transplant marrow is not evident post-transplant. Chromosomal analysis showed a normal karyotype in all 20 cells, and chimerism studies showed 100% donor origin.

Other Reactive Conditions

Expansion of non-classical monocytes (CD14 lo/CD16+) in peripheral blood has been reported in various inflammatory or infections conditions, such as rheumatoid arthritis, hemodialysis, hypercholesterolemia, Kawasaki disease, and bacterial and viral infections.[107] In comparison to classical monocytes, non-classical monocytes express CD16 and decreased levels of CD14, CD15, CD33, CD38, and CD64.[107] Despite decreased CD14, these non-classical monocytes are a subset of mature monocytes and should not be confused for immature monocytic cells.

An increased percentage of CD14 bright/CD56+ monocytes in peripheral blood has been described in autoimmune diseases. In patients with active Crohn's disease, the percentage of CD56+ monocytes is significantly increased compared with the controls.[108] Similarly, in patients with rheumatoid arthritis, the frequency of CD56+ monocytes was significantly higher than in healthy controls and this difference was more prominent in patients younger than 40 years of age, with possible contribution to inflammatory response.[109]

CD64 is expressed at a low level on neutrophils in a resting state. In patients with systemic infection and sepsis, CD64 expression significantly increases on neutrophils, and as well on monocytes thought the impact is less pronounced.[17,110]

After moderate to high intensity exercise and severe traumatic injury, CD16 expression on neutrophils was reduced; neutrophil degranulation and respiratory burst activity were maintained.[111,112] Besides MDS, decreased CD10 expression on neutrophils may been seen in HIV-positive patients and septic shock.[113,114] One additional technical consideration to keep in mind when evaluating CD16 on neutrophils is specimen viability as CD16 expression on mature apoptotic neutrophils may be reduced.[115]

FLOW CYTOMETRY IN THE DIAGNOSTIC WORK UP OF MYELODYSPLASTIC SYNDROMES/NEOPLASMS

Although MFC alone is not sufficient to establish a primary diagnosis of MDS, a number of previous and more recent studies have shown that MFC can aid the diagnosis and prognostication of patients with MDS. However, implementation of MFC into routine clinical practices with appropriate standardization is challenging due to lack of consensus on pre-analytical procedures, data analysis, data interpretation, and reporting.

Current Recommendations

ELN/iMDS Flow has recently published updated recommendations for the application of MFC in the diagnosis of MDS.[34,116–118] These include recommendations for pre-analytical and technical issues including optimal methods of sample processing, antibody panels, and hardware[118]; analytical issues including analysis of myeloid precursors, maturing granulocytic and monocytic cells, and erythroid precursors[34]; and discussion of the rationale of incorporating MFC in the diagnostic work up of cytopenia and suspected MDS.[117] These detailed recommendations will facilitate the appropriate implementation of MFC assay across different laboratories.

Diagnostic Multiparametric Flow Cytometry Scoring Systems in the Diagnosis of Myelodysplastic Syndromes/Neoplasms

Current data suggest that aberrancy of a single antigen is not sufficiently specific in distinguishing normal from dysplastic populations and should not be interpreted as evidence of MDS when present in isolation. Most investigators have demonstrated that an increase in the number of abnormalities detected increases specificity for MDS. In an effort to standardize and enumerate flow cytometric abnormalities in MDS, several MFC scoring systems that quantify the number and severity of immunophenotypic aberrancies in different lineages using different panels have been proposed and validated, allowing efficient discrimination of MDS from normal/reactive conditions. Two recent studies compared diagnostic power and prognostic impact of several widely used scoring systems. One prospective study compared flow cytometric scoring system (FCSS) score,[45,119] Ogata score,[1,2] Red-score,[74] European Leukemia Net - nucleated erythroid cells (ELN-NEC) score,[76] and integrated flow cytometric score (iFS) score[61] in discriminating MDS from non-clonal cytopenias and healthy bone marrow. The iFS score, which is the most comprehensive and includes 44 parameters, showed the highest accuracy and well-balanced sensitivity and specificity in diagnosing MDS.[37] Furthermore, a designation of "consistent with MDS" as defined by iFS was significantly associated with an inferior survival, emphasizing the prognostic relevance of MFC scores. The second study compared Ogata score, Wells score (FCSS), and iFS score in separating MDS, cytopenias without myeloid disorder and healthy donors.[120] The results also confirmed that iFS is the most preferred MFC scoring system in diagnosing MDS.[120] It is possible that the relatively high number of parameters included in the iFS score render it somewhat challenging for many laboratories to employ, in particular, when using manual analysis strategies. Additionally, to date, there has been no larger multicenter study that uses a harmonized gating/analysis protocol covering all the parameters included in the iFS.

SUMMARY

MFC is a valuable ancillary tool in the evaluation of patients with suspected MDS. Multiple studies have demonstrated the clinical utility of MFC in the diagnosis, classification, and prognostication of MDS. Evaluation of a combination of antigens across various cellular populations for assessment of maturational patterns is necessary to distinguish reactive aberrancies from MDS associated abnormalities. Given the numbers of parameters assessed and complexity of data analysis, accurate application of this testing modality requires experience and standardization of all phases of testing including the pre-analytic phase, panel design, instrumentation, data analysis, interpretation, and reporting. MFC is known to provide excellent analyst concordance where harmonized analysis protocols are used.[43] Furthermore, interinterpreter and interlaboratory variation can be reduced with experience and a coordinated approach.[121] Such challenges in standardization have contributed to the delayed widespread adoption of this testing modality; however, is possible that MDS analysis by MFC may be more easily incorporated by a larger number of laboratories if an established and harmonized protocol is available. Further gains may be added with introduction and implementation of automated data analysis strategies. Although not yet clinically accredited, a novel computational diagnostic workflow including pre-processing MFC data, dimensionality reductions, and clustering methods to detect a cell population (FlowSOM), with implementation of a machine learning classifier to identify MDS has recently been described and tested. This approach outperformed conventional MFC scores with respect to diagnostic accuracy and efficiency.[122] In the future, such automated diagnostic tools may facilitate and improve data analysis in the clinical setting, and contribute to more uniform and standardized data sets for accurate diagnosis, bringing MFC for MDS into mainstream laboratory use.

CLINICS CARE POINTS

- Multiparametric flow cytometry (MFC) is a useful tool in evaluating patients with myelodysplastic syndromes/neoplasms (MDS).

- Normal maturation is accompanied by conserved changes in antigen expression with maturation. MFC for MDS is grounded in demonstrating deviations from normal patterns of antigen expression.

- Immunophenotypic abnormalities may be demonstrated on progenitors and differentiating cells of lineages including myeloid, monocytic, and erythroid lineages.

- MFC should be used in conjunction with clinical data, morphology, and genetic data to arrive and a definitive diagnosis of MDS and for specific classification.

- Reactive changes can be accompanied by shifts in antigen expression that should not be mistaken for dysplasia.

CONFLICT OF INTEREST STATEMENT

All authors declare that they have no conflict of interest.

REFERENCES

1. Della Porta MG, Picone C, Pascutto C, et al. Multicenter validation of a reproducible flow cytometric score for the diagnosis of low-grade myelodysplastic syndromes: results of a European LeukemiaNET study. Haematologica 2012; 97(8):1209–17.
2. Ogata K, Della Porta MG, Malcovati L, et al. Diagnostic utility of flow cytometry in low-grade myelodysplastic syndromes: a prospective validation study. Haematologica 2009;94(8):1066–74.
3. Wood BL. Myeloid malignancies: myelodysplastic syndromes, myeloproliferative disorders, and acute myeloid leukemia. Clin Lab Med 2007;27(3):551–75, vii.
4. Arnoulet C, Bene MC, Durrieu F, et al. Four- and five-color flow cytometry analysis of leukocyte differentiation pathways in normal bone marrow: a reference document based on a systematic approach by the GTLLF and GEIL. Cytometry B Clin Cytom 2010;78(1):4–10.
5. Gorczyca W, Sun ZY, Cronin W, et al. Immunophenotypic pattern of myeloid populations by flow cytometry analysis. Methods Cell Biol 2011;103:221–66.
6. Stelzer GT, Shults KE, Loken MR. CD45 gating for routine flow cytometric analysis of human bone marrow specimens. Ann N Y Acad Sci 1993;677:265–80.
7. Terstappen LW, Safford M, Loken MR. Flow cytometric analysis of human bone marrow. III. Neutrophil maturation. Leukemia 1990;4(9):657–63.
8. Barreau S, Green AS, Dussiau C, et al. Phenotypic landscape of granulocytes and monocytes by multiparametric flow cytometry: a prospective study of a 1-tube panel strategy for diagnosis and prognosis of patients with MDS. Cytometry B Clin Cytom 2020;98(3):226–37.
9. Fajtova M, Kovarikova A, Svec P, et al. Immunophenotypic profile of nucleated erythroid progenitors during maturation in regenerating bone marrow. Leuk Lymphoma 2013;54(11):2523–30.
10. Machherndl-Spandl S, Suessner S, Danzer M, et al. Molecular pathways of early CD105-positive erythroid cells as compared with CD34-positive common precursor cells by flow cytometric cell-sorting and gene expression profiling. Blood Cancer J 2013;3(1):e100.

11. Wangen JR, Eidenschink Brodersen L, Stolk TT, et al. Assessment of normal erythropoiesis by flow cytometry: important considerations for specimen preparation. Int J Lab Hematol 2014;36(2):184–96.

12. Borowitz MJ, Guenther KL, Shults KE, et al. Immunophenotyping of acute leukemia by flow cytometric analysis. Use of CD45 and right-angle light scatter to gate on leukemic blasts in three-color analysis. Am J Clin Pathol 1993;100(5):534–40.

13. Jacobsen SEW, Nerlov C. Haematopoiesis in the era of advanced single-cell technologies. Nat Cell Biol 2019;21(1):2–8.

14. Manz MG, Miyamoto T, Akashi K, et al. Prospective isolation of human clonogenic common myeloid progenitors. Proc Natl Acad Sci U S A 2002;99(18):11872–7.

15. Ratajczak MZ. Phenotypic and functional characterization of hematopoietic stem cells. Curr Opin Hematol 2008;15(4):293–300.

16. Kussick SJ, Wood BL. Using 4-color flow cytometry to identify abnormal myeloid populations. Arch Pathol Lab Med 2003;127(9):1140–7.

17. Davis BH, Olsen SH, Ahmad E, et al. Neutrophil CD64 is an improved indicator of infection or sepsis in emergency department patients. Arch Pathol Lab Med 2006;130(5):654–61.

18. Terstappen LW, Hollander Z, Meiners H, et al. Quantitative comparison of myeloid antigens on five lineages of mature peripheral blood cells. J Leukoc Biol 1990;48(2):138–48.

19. Yang DT, Greenwood JH, Hartung L, et al. Flow cytometric analysis of different CD14 epitopes can help identify immature monocytic populations. Am J Clin Pathol 2005;124(6):930–6.

20. Fattizzo B, Ireland R, Dunlop A, et al. Clinical and prognostic significance of small paroxysmal nocturnal hemoglobinuria clones in myelodysplastic syndrome and aplastic anemia. Leukemia 2021;35(11):3223–31.

21. Wang SA, Pozdnyakova O, Jorgensen JL, et al. Detection of paroxysmal nocturnal hemoglobinuria clones in patients with myelodysplastic syndromes and related bone marrow diseases, with emphasis on diagnostic pitfalls and caveats. Haematologica 2009;94(1):29–37.

22. Boyette LB, Macedo C, Hadi K, et al. Phenotype, function, and differentiation potential of human monocyte subsets. PLoS One 2017;12(4):e0176460.

23. Matarraz S, Almeida J, Flores-Montero J, et al. Introduction to the diagnosis and classification of monocytic-lineage leukemias by flow cytometry. Cytometry B Clin Cytom 2017;92(3):218–27.

24. Orfao A, Matarraz S, Perez-Andres M, et al. EuroFlow. Immunophenotypic dissection of normal hematopoiesis. J Immunol Methods 2019;475:112684.

25. Bene MC, Axler O, Violidaki D, et al. Definition of erythroid differentiation subsets in normal human bone marrow using FlowSOM Unsupervised cluster analysis of flow cytometry data. Hemasphere 2021;5(1):e512.

26. Kalina T, Flores-Montero J, van der Velden VH, et al. EuroFlow standardization of flow cytometer instrument settings and immunophenotyping protocols. Leukemia 2012;26(9):1986–2010.

27. Mello FV, Land MGP, Costa ES, et al. Maturation-associated gene expression profiles during normal human bone marrow erythropoiesis. Cell Death Discov 2019;5:69.

28. Mirabelli P, Di Noto R, Lo Pardo C, et al. Extended flow cytometry characterization of normal bone marrow progenitor cells by simultaneous detection of

aldehyde dehydrogenase and early hematopoietic antigens: implication for erythroid differentiation studies. BMC Physiol 2008;8:13.

29. Fang H, Wang SA, You MJ, et al. Flow cytometry immunophenotypic features of pure erythroid leukemia and the distinction from reactive erythroid precursors. Cytometry B Clin Cytom 2022;102(6):440–7.

30. Porwit A, Violidaki D, Axler O, et al. Unsupervised cluster analysis and subset characterization of abnormal erythropoiesis using the bioinformatic Flow-Self Organizing Maps algorithm. Cytometry B Clin Cytom 2022;102(2):134–42.

31. Violidaki D, Axler O, Jafari K, et al. Analysis of erythroid maturation in the non-lysed bone marrow with help of radar plots facilitates detection of flow cytometric aberrations in myelodysplastic syndromes. Cytometry B Clin Cytom 2020; 98(5):399–411.

32. Yan H, Ali A, Blanc L, et al. Comprehensive phenotyping of erythropoiesis in human bone marrow: evaluation of normal and ineffective erythropoiesis. Am J Hematol 2021;96(9):1064–76.

33. Sutherland DR, Illingworth A, Marinov I, et al. ICCS/ESCCA consensus guidelines to detect GPI-deficient cells in paroxysmal nocturnal hemoglobinuria (PNH) and related disorders part 2 - reagent selection and assay optimization for high-sensitivity testing. Cytometry B Clin Cytom 2018;94(1):23–48.

34. Porwit A, Bene MC, Duetz C, et al. Multiparameter flow cytometry in the evaluation of myelodysplasia: analytical issues: recommendations from the European LeukemiaNet/international myelodysplastic syndrome flow cytometry working group. Cytometry B Clin Cytom 2023;104(1):27–50.

35. Allan RW, Ansari-Lari MA, Jordan S. DRAQ5-based, no-lyse, no-wash bone marrow aspirate evaluation by flow cytometry. Am J Clin Pathol 2008;129(5): 706–13.

36. Swerdlow SH, Campo E, Harris NL, et al. WHO classification of Tumours of Haematopoietic and lymphoid Tissues. Revised 4th Edition ed. Lyon: International Agency for Research on Cancer; 2017.

37. Oelschlaegel U, Oelschlaeger L, von Bonin M, et al. Comparison of five diagnostic flow cytometry scores in patients with myelodysplastic syndromes: diagnostic power and prognostic impact. Cytometry B Clin Cytom 2021;104(2): 141–50.

38. Kern W, Westers TM, Bellos F, et al. Multicenter prospective evaluation of diagnostic potential of flow cytometric aberrancies in myelodysplastic syndromes by the ELN iMDS flow working group. Cytometry B Clin Cytom 2023;104(1):51–65.

39. Matarraz S, Lopez A, Barrena S, et al. Bone marrow cells from myelodysplastic syndromes show altered immunophenotypic profiles that may contribute to the diagnosis and prognostic stratification of the disease: a pilot study on a series of 56 patients. Cytometry B Clin Cytom 2010;78(3):154–68.

40. Xu F, Guo J, Wu LY, et al. Diagnostic application and clinical significance of FCM progress scoring system based on immunophenotyping in CD34+ blasts in myelodysplastic syndromes. Cytometry B Clin Cytom 2013;84(4):267–78.

41. Chen X, Fromm JR, Naresh KN. "Blasts" in myeloid neoplasms - how do we define blasts and how do we incorporate them into diagnostic schema moving forward? Leukemia 2022;36(2):327–32.

42. Hodes A, Calvo KR, Dulau A, et al. The challenging task of enumerating blasts in the bone marrow. Semin Hematol 2019;56(1):58–64.

43. Johansson U, McIver-Brown N, Cullen M, et al. The flow cytometry myeloid progenitor count: a reproducible parameter for diagnosis and prognosis of myelodysplastic syndromes. Cytometry B Clin Cytom 2023;104(2):115–27.

44. Ogata K, Kishikawa Y, Satoh C, et al. Diagnostic application of flow cytometric characteristics of CD34+ cells in low-grade myelodysplastic syndromes. Blood 2006;108(3):1037–44.
45. Wells DA, Benesch M, Loken MR, et al. Myeloid and monocytic dyspoiesis as determined by flow cytometric scoring in myelodysplastic syndrome correlates with the IPSS and with outcome after hematopoietic stem cell transplantation. Blood 2003;102(1):394–403.
46. Kussick SJ, Fromm JR, Rossini A, et al. Four-color flow cytometry shows strong concordance with bone marrow morphology and cytogenetics in the evaluation for myelodysplasia. Am J Clin Pathol 2005;124(2):170–81.
47. da Silva-Coelho P, Kroeze LI, Yoshida K, et al. Clonal evolution in myelodysplastic syndromes. Nat Commun 2017;8:15099.
48. Woll PS, Kjallquist U, Chowdhury O, et al. Myelodysplastic syndromes are propagated by rare and distinct human cancer stem cells in vivo. Cancer Cell 2014; 25(6):794–808.
49. Stevens BM, Khan N, D'Alessandro A, et al. Characterization and targeting of malignant stem cells in patients with advanced myelodysplastic syndromes. Nat Commun 2018;9(1):3694.
50. Pang WW, Pluvinage JV, Price EA, et al. Hematopoietic stem cell and progenitor cell mechanisms in myelodysplastic syndromes. Proc Natl Acad Sci U S A 2013; 110(8):3011–6.
51. Will B, Zhou L, Vogler TO, et al. Stem and progenitor cells in myelodysplastic syndromes show aberrant stage-specific expansion and harbor genetic and epigenetic alterations. Blood 2012;120(10):2076–86.
52. Tehranchi R, Woll PS, Anderson K, et al. Persistent malignant stem cells in del(5q) myelodysplasia in remission. N Engl J Med 2010;363(11):1025–37.
53. Shameli A, Dharmani-Khan P, Luider J, et al. Exploring blast composition in myelodysplastic syndromes and myelodysplastic/myeloproliferative neoplasms: CD45RA and CD371 improve diagnostic value of flow cytometry through assessment of myeloblast heterogeneity and stem cell aberrancy. Cytometry B Clin Cytom 2021;100(5):574–89.
54. Majeti R, Park CY, Weissman IL. Identification of a hierarchy of multipotent hematopoietic progenitors in human cord blood. Cell Stem Cell 2007;1(6):635–45.
55. Li LJ, Tao JL, Fu R, et al. Increased CD34+CD38 -CD123 + cells in myelodysplastic syndrome displaying malignant features similar to those in AML. Int J Hematol 2014;100(1):60–9.
56. Ostendorf BN, Flenner E, Florcken A, et al. Phenotypic characterization of aberrant stem and progenitor cell populations in myelodysplastic syndromes. PLoS One 2018;13(5):e0197823.
57. Della Porta MG, Picone C, Tenore A, et al. Prognostic significance of reproducible immunophenotypic markers of marrow dysplasia. Haematologica 2014; 99(1):e8–10.
58. Stetler-Stevenson M, Arthur DC, Jabbour N, et al. Diagnostic utility of flow cytometric immunophenotyping in myelodysplastic syndrome. Blood 2001;98(4): 979–87.
59. van de Loosdrecht AA, Ireland R, Kern W, et al. Rationale for the clinical application of flow cytometry in patients with myelodysplastic syndromes: position paper of an International Consortium and the European LeukemiaNet Working Group. Leuk Lymphoma 2013;54(3):472–5.

60. Duetz C, Westers TM, van de Loosdrecht AA. Clinical implication of multi-parameter flow cytometry in myelodysplastic syndromes. Pathobiology 2019; 86(1):14–23.

61. Cremers EM, Westers TM, Alhan C, et al. Implementation of erythroid lineage analysis by flow cytometry in diagnostic models for myelodysplastic syndromes. Haematologica 2017;102(2):320–6.

62. Kern W, Haferlach C, Schnittger S, et al. Clinical utility of multiparameter flow cytometry in the diagnosis of 1013 patients with suspected myelodysplastic syndrome: correlation to cytomorphology, cytogenetics, and clinical data. Cancer 2010;116(19):4549–63.

63. Chen X, Wood BL, Cherian S. Immunophenotypic features of myeloid neoplasms associated with chromosome 7 abnormalities. Cytometry B Clin Cytom 2019;96(4):300–9.

64. Westers TM, Ireland R, Kern W, et al. Standardization of flow cytometry in myelodysplastic syndromes: a report from an international consortium and the European LeukemiaNet Working Group. Leukemia 2012;26(7):1730–41.

65. Harrington AM, Schelling LA, Ordobazari A, et al. Immunophenotypes of chronic myelomonocytic leukemia (CMML) subtypes by flow cytometry: a comparison of CMML-1 vs CMML-2, myeloproliferative vs dysplastic, De Novo vs therapy-related, and CMML-specific cytogenetic risk subtypes. Am J Clin Pathol 2016; 146(2):170–81.

66. Wu A, Gao P, Wu N, et al. Elevated mature monocytes in bone marrow accompanied with a higher IPSS-R score predicts a poor prognosis in myelodysplastic syndromes. BMC Cancer 2021;21(1):546.

67. van de Loosdrecht AA, Alhan C, Bene MC, et al. Standardization of flow cytometry in myelodysplastic syndromes: report from the first European LeukemiaNet working conference on flow cytometry in myelodysplastic syndromes. Haematologica 2009;94(8):1124–34.

68. Lambert C, Preijers F, Yanikkaya Demirel G, et al. Monocytes and macrophages in flow: an ESCCA initiative on advanced analyses of monocyte lineage using flow cytometry. Cytometry B Clin Cytom 2017;92(3):180–8.

69. Patnaik MM, Timm MM, Vallapureddy R, et al. Flow cytometry based monocyte subset analysis accurately distinguishes chronic myelomonocytic leukemia from myeloproliferative neoplasms with associated monocytosis. Blood Cancer J 2017;7(7):e584.

70. Selimoglu-Buet D, Wagner-Ballon O, Saada V, et al. Characteristic repartition of monocyte subsets as a diagnostic signature of chronic myelomonocytic leukemia. Blood 2015;125(23):3618–26.

71. Tarfi S, Harrivel V, Dumezy F, et al. Groupe Francophone des, M. Multicenter validation of the flow measurement of classical monocyte fraction for chronic myelomonocytic leukemia diagnosis. Blood Cancer J 2018;8(11):114.

72. Wagner-Ballon O, Bettelheim P, Lauf J, et al. European LeukemiaNet International, M. D. S. F. C. W. G. ELN iMDS flow working group validation of the monocyte assay for chronic myelomonocytic leukemia diagnosis by flow cytometry. Cytometry B Clin Cytom 2023;104(1):66–76.

73. Eidenschink Brodersen L, Menssen AJ, Wangen JR, et al. Assessment of erythroid dysplasia by "difference from normal" in routine clinical flow cytometry workup. Cytometry B Clin Cytom 2015;88(2):125–35.

74. Mathis S, Chapuis N, Debord C, et al. Flow cytometric detection of dyserythropoiesis: a sensitive and powerful diagnostic tool for myelodysplastic syndromes. Leukemia 2013;27(10):1981–7.

75. Malcovati L, Della Porta MG, Lunghi M, et al. Flow cytometry evaluation of erythroid and myeloid dysplasia in patients with myelodysplastic syndrome. Leukemia 2005;19(5):776–83.
76. Westers TM, Cremers EM, Oelschlaegel U, et al. Immunophenotypic analysis of erythroid dysplasia in myelodysplastic syndromes. A report from the IMDSFlow working group. Haematologica 2017;102(2):308–19.
77. Johansson U, Rolf N, Futhee N, et al. Erythroid side scatter: a parameter that improves diagnostic accuracy of flow cytometry myelodysplastic syndrome scoring. Cytometry B Clin Cytom 2023;104(2):151–61.
78. Duetz C, Westers TM, In 't Hout FEM, et al. Distinct bone marrow immunophenotypic features define the splicing factor 3B subunit 1 (SF3B1)-mutant myelodysplastic syndromes subtype. Br J Haematol 2021;193(4):798–803.
79. Fang H, Wang SA, Hu S, et al. Acute promyelocytic leukemia: immunophenotype and differential diagnosis by flow cytometry. Cytometry B Clin Cytom 2022;102(4):283–91.
80. Arana Rosainz MJ, Nguyen N, Wahed A, et al. Acute myeloid leukemia with mutated NPM1 mimics acute promyelocytic leukemia presentation. Int J Lab Hematol 2021;43(2):218–26.
81. Albano F, Mestice A, Pannunzio A, et al. The biological characteristics of CD34+ CD2+ adult acute promyelocytic leukemia and the CD34 CD2 hypergranular (M3) and microgranular (M3v) phenotypes. Haematologica 2006;91(3):311–6.
82. Gupta M, Jafari K, Rajab A, et al. Radar plots facilitate differential diagnosis of acute promyelocytic leukemia and NPM1+ acute myeloid leukemia by flow cytometry. Cytometry B Clin Cytom 2021;100(4):409–20.
83. Orfao A, Chillon MC, Bortoluci AM, et al. The flow cytometric pattern of CD34, CD15 and CD13 expression in acute myeloblastic leukemia is highly characteristic of the presence of PML-RARalpha gene rearrangements. Haematologica 1999;84(5):405–12.
84. De J, Zanjani R, Hibbard M, et al. Immunophenotypic profile predictive of KIT activating mutations in AML1-ETO leukemia. Am J Clin Pathol 2007;128(4):550–7.
85. Khoury H, Dalal BI, Nantel SH, et al. Correlation between karyotype and quantitative immunophenotype in acute myelogenous leukemia with t(8;21). Mod Pathol 2004;17(10):1211–6.
86. Khoury H, Dalal BI, Nevill TJ, et al. Acute myelogenous leukemia with t(8;21)–identification of a specific immunophenotype. Leuk Lymphoma 2003;44(10):1713–8.
87. Angelini DF, Ottone T, Guerrera G, et al. A leukemia-associated CD34/CD123/CD25/CD99+ immunophenotype Identifies FLT3-mutated clones in acute myeloid leukemia. Clin Cancer Res 2015;21(17):3977–85.
88. Kussick SJ, Stirewalt DL, Yi HS, et al. A distinctive nuclear morphology in acute myeloid leukemia is strongly associated with loss of HLA-DR expression and FLT3 internal tandem duplication. Leukemia 2004;18(10):1591–8.
89. Zhou Y, Moon A, Hoyle E, et al. Pattern associated leukemia immunophenotypes and measurable disease detection in acute myeloid leukemia or myelodysplastic syndrome with mutated NPM1. Cytometry B Clin Cytom 2019;96(1):67–72.
90. Greenberg PL, Tuechler H, Schanz J, et al. Revised international prognostic scoring system for myelodysplastic syndromes. Blood 2012;120(12):2454–65.
91. Khoury JD, Solary E, Abla O, et al. The 5th edition of the World Health Organization classification of Haematolymphoid Tumours: myeloid and Histiocytic/dendritic neoplasms. Leukemia 2022;36(7):1703–19.

92. Arber DA, Orazi A, Hasserjian RP, et al. International consensus classification of myeloid neoplasms and acute leukemias: integrating morphologic, clinical, and genomic data. Blood 2022;140(11):1200–28.

93. Oelschlaegel U, Westers TM, Mohr B, et al. Myelodysplastic syndromes with a deletion 5q display a characteristic immunophenotypic profile suitable for diagnostics and response monitoring. Haematologica 2015;100(3):e93–6.

94. Papaemmanuil E, Gerstung M, Malcovati L, et al. Clinical and biological implications of driver mutations in myelodysplastic syndromes. Blood 2013;122(22): 3616–27, quiz 3699.

95. Muroi K, Fujiwara S, Tatara R, et al. CD56 expression in normal immature granulocytes after allogeneic hematopoietic stem cell transplantation. J Clin Exp Hematop 2013;53(3):247–50.

96. Carulli G. Effects of recombinant human granulocyte colony-stimulating factor administration on neutrophil phenotype and functions. Haematologica 1997; 82(5):606–16.

97. Illingworth AJ, Marinov I, Sutherland DR. Sensitive and accurate identification of PNH clones based on ICCS/ESCCA PNH Consensus Guidelines-A summary. Int J Lab Hematol 2019;41(Suppl 1):73–81.

98. de Haas M. IgG-Fc receptors and the clinical relevance of their polymorphisms. Wien Klin Wochenschr 2001;113(20–21):825–31.

99. de Haas M, Kleijer M, van Zwieten R, et al. Neutrophil Fc gamma RIIIb deficiency, nature, and clinical consequences: a study of 21 individuals from 14 families. Blood 1995;86(6):2403–13.

100. Tamm A, Schmidt RE. The binding epitopes of human CD16 (Fc gamma RIII) monoclonal antibodies. Implications for ligand binding. J Immunol 1996; 157(4):1576–81.

101. Costello C. An update on the role of daratumumab in the treatment of multiple myeloma. Ther Adv Hematol 2017;8(1):28–37.

102. Oberle A, Brandt A, Alawi M, et al. Long-term CD38 saturation by daratumumab interferes with diagnostic myeloma cell detection. Haematologica 2017;102(9): e368–70.

103. Gadgeel M, AlQanber B, Buck S, et al. Aberrant myelomonocytic CD56 expression in Down syndrome is frequent and not associated with leukemogenesis. Ann Hematol 2021;100(7):1695–700.

104. Langebrake C, Klusmann JH, Wortmann K, et al. Concomitant aberrant overexpression of RUNX1 and NCAM in regenerating bone marrow of myeloid leukemia of Down's syndrome. Haematologica 2006;91(11):1473–80.

105. Karandikar NJ, Aquino DB, McKenna RW, et al. Transient myeloproliferative disorder and acute myeloid leukemia in Down syndrome. An immunophenotypic analysis. Am J Clin Pathol 2001;116(2):204–10.

106. Hsu FC, Hudson C, Wilson ER, et al. The impact of Down syndrome-specific non-malignant hematopoietic regeneration in the bone marrow on the detection of leukemic measurable residual disease. Cytometry B Clin Cytom 2023. https://doi.org/10.1002/cyto.b.22118.

107. Ziegler-Heitbrock L. The CD14+ CD16+ blood monocytes: their role in infection and inflammation. J Leukoc Biol 2007;81(3):584–92.

108. Grip O, Bredberg A, Lindgren S, et al. Increased subpopulations of CD16(+) and CD56(+) blood monocytes in patients with active Crohn's disease. Inflamm Bowel Dis 2007;13(5):566–72.

109. Krasselt M, Baerwald C, Wagner U, et al. CD56+ monocytes have a dysregu-lated cytokine response to lipopolysaccharide and accumulate in rheumatoid arthritis and immunosenescence. Arthritis Res Ther 2013;15(5):R139.

110. Hoffmann JJ. Neutrophil CD64: a diagnostic marker for infection and sepsis. Clin Chem Lab Med 2009;47(8):903–16.

111. Peake J, Wilson G, Hordern M, et al. Changes in neutrophil surface receptor expression, degranulation, and respiratory burst activity after moderate- and high-intensity exercise. J Appl Physiol (1985) 2004;97(2):612–8.

112. White-Owen C, Alexander JW, Babcock GF. Reduced expression of neutrophil CD11b and CD16 after severe traumatic injury. J Surg Res 1992;52(1):22–6.

113. Martens A, Eppink GJ, Woittiez AJ, et al. Neutrophil function capacity to express CD10 is decreased in patients with septic shock. Crit Care Med 1999;27(3): 549–53.

114. van de Vyver A, Delport E, Visser A. Decreased CD10 expression in the bone marrow neutrophils of HIV positive patients. Mediterr J Hematol Infect Dis 2010;2(3):e2010032.

115. Dransfield I, Buckle AM, Savill JS, et al. Neutrophil apoptosis is associated with a reduction in CD16 (Fc gamma RIII) expression. J Immunol 1994;153(3):1254–63.

116. Porwit A, van de Loosdrecht AA, Bettelheim P, et al. Revisiting guidelines for integration of flow cytometry results in the WHO classification of myelodysplastic syndromes-proposal from the International/European LeukemiaNet Working Group for Flow Cytometry in MDS. Leukemia 2014;28(9):1793–8.

117. van de Loosdrecht AA, Kern W, Porwit A, et al. Clinical application of flow cytom-etry in patients with unexplained cytopenia and suspected myelodysplastic syn-drome: a report of the European LeukemiaNet International MDS-Flow Cytometry Working Group. Cytometry B Clin Cytom 2023;104(1):77–86.

118. van der Velden VHJ, Preijers F, Johansson U, et al. Flow cytometric analysis of myelodysplasia: pre-analytical and technical issues-Recommendations from the European LeukemiaNet. Cytometry B Clin Cytom 2023;104(1):15–26.

119. Alhan C, Westers TM, Cremers EM, et al. High flow cytometric scores identify adverse prognostic subgroups within the revised international prognostic scoring system for myelodysplastic syndromes. Br J Haematol 2014;167(1): 100–9.

120. Davydova YO, Parovichnikova EN, Galtseva IV, et al. Diagnostic significance of flow cytometry scales in diagnostics of myelodysplastic syndromes. Cytometry B Clin Cytom 2021;100(3):312–21.

121. Westers TM, van der Velden VH, Alhan C, et al, Working Party on Flow Cytom-etry in, M. D. S. o. D. S. o. C. Implementation of flow cytometry in the diagnostic work-up of myelodysplastic syndromes in a multicenter approach: report from the Dutch Working Party on Flow Cytometry in MDS. Leuk Res 2012;36(4): 422–30.

122. Duetz C, Van Gassen S, Westers TM, et al. Computational flow cytometry as a diagnostic tool in suspected-myelodysplastic syndromes. Cytometry 2021; 99(8):814–24.

Molecular Techniques and Gene Mutations in Myelodysplastic Syndromes

Hadrian Mendoza, MD[a], Alexa J. Siddon, MD[b,c],*

KEYWORDS

- Mutations • Myelodysplastic syndromes • Myelodysplasia
- Next-generation sequencing • Whole-genome sequencing

KEY POINTS

- Myelodysplastic syndromes (MDS) are increasingly understood to be a genetically defined disease.
- Gene mutations now define several subclassifications of MDS based on the most current classification systems.
- Gene mutations are present in most cases of MDS and often have prognostic and clinical implications.
- Advances in DNA sequencing technology allow for greater personalization in the diagnosis and management of MDS.
- Efforts are underway to incorporate into clinical practice a standardized MDS risk assessment tool that includes molecular data.

INTRODUCTION

Myelodysplastic syndromes (MDSs), now also referred to as myelodysplastic neoplasms,[1] are a biologically and clinically diverse group of hematologic malignancies characterized by morphologic dysplasia, peripheral cytopenias, and potential transformation to acute myeloid leukemia (AML). Two recent revisions to the classification system of MDS: one, the World Health Organization Classification of Haematolymphoid Tumors (WHO-HAEM5), and the other by the Society for Hematopathology and the European Association for Haematopathology forming a Clinical Advisory Committee, which resulted in the International Consensus Classification (ICC), highlight the increasing understanding of MDS as a genetically defined disease, a change

[a] Department of Internal Medicine, Yale School of Medicine, PO Box 208030, New Haven, CT 06520, USA; [b] Department of Laboratory Medicine, Yale School of Medicine, New Haven, CT, USA; [c] Department of Pathology, Yale School of Medicine, New Haven, CT, USA
* Corresponding author. Department of Laboratory Medicine, Yale School of Medicine, 330 Cedar Street, PO Box 208035, New Haven, CT 06520.
E-mail address: alexa.siddon@yale.edu

Clin Lab Med 43 (2023) 549–563
https://doi.org/10.1016/j.cll.2023.06.002
0272-2712/23/© 2023 Elsevier Inc. All rights reserved.
labmed.theclinics.com

from previous systems in which MDS was classified by morphologic findings or risk of progression to AML.[1,2] Genetic lesions in MDS may be inherited, arise spontaneously, or be induced by environmental exposures including cytotoxic chemotherapy and radiotherapy.[3] At times, they carry prognostic and clinical significance, guide selection of targeted antineoplastic agents, facilitate risk stratification, and may be used to monitor residual disease after initial treatment.[4] Although MDS is most common in older adults (median age at diagnosis of 77 years), it can arise at any age.[5] Detailed discussion of germline mutations and childhood MDS (also known as refractory cytopenia of childhood) can be found in other articles in this review series. The present discussion focuses primarily on acquired genetic mutations associated with adult MDS.

MOLECULAR TESTING IN MYELODYSPLASTIC SYNDROME

The initial assessment of a patient with suspected MDS includes a complete blood count; peripheral blood smear; and bone marrow evaluation including morphologic assessment, immunohistochemistry, cytogenetic analysis, and molecular testing, with or without multiparameter flow cytometry (MFC). Methods of cytogenetic analysis for chromosomal abnormalities include karyotyping, fluorescence in situ hybridization (FISH), and chromosomal microarrays (CMAs), whereas testing for specific gene mutations traditionally includes Sanger sequencing and polymerase chain reaction (PCR), with next-generation sequencing (NGS) taking an increasingly important role.[6]

Cytogenetic Analysis

Karyotyping (ie, chromosome banding) is the oldest and most used method to assess for chromosomal aberrations including copy number and structural abnormalities due to its wide availability and high success rate that has been demonstrated since the 1980s.[7,8] It is limited by poor resolution in detecting abnormalities smaller than 10 Mbases, low analytical sensitivity of 10^{-1} (abnormalities present in 5%–10% of cells), and the need to analyze cultured cells dividing in vitro, as obtaining sufficient metaphase cells in culture is not always feasible in certain hematologic malignancies.[7,9] Turnaround time may be as quick as 48 hours but more typically take 2 to 3 weeks, depending on individual laboratory practices.[6]

FISH overcomes the requirement to use cultured dividing cells, as it can be used on fixed or interphase cells. It exhibits greater analytical sensitivity (10^{-2}; abnormalities present in 1%–5% of cells) than karyotyping and has higher resolution to detect gene-level chromosomal abnormalities missed by conventional karyotyping,[10,11] though in one study of 544 bone marrow specimens obtained for diagnosis and 364 specimens obtained for follow-up of MDS, karyotype and FISH were concordant 98.3% of the time at diagnosis and 97% of the time at follow-up.[12] Whereas karyotyping allows for assessment of the whole genome, FISH probes must be targeted toward a gene or region of interest and limit most clinical laboratories to the use of commercially available probes.[7,13] It is typically faster than karyotyping, usually completed within 1 to 3 days.[6]

CMAs do not require cultured cells and exhibit enhanced resolution (around 25–50 Kbases) to detect unbalanced abnormalities compared with karyotyping. In addition, they can visualize copy number-neutral loss of heterozygosity, which is not seen on karyotyping.[14] CMAs offer an advantage over FISH in that they do not require targeted probes and can detect abnormalities across the genome in an unbiased approach.[6] They are limited by poorer analytical sensitivity compared with karyotype and FISH (>10^{-1}; abnormalities present in 20%–30% of cells), the inability to detect balanced rearrangements commonly found in hematologic malignancies, and higher cost.[6,7]

Turnaround time for CMAs is typically longer than FISH or karyotyping, ranging from 3 to 14 days, and may not be routinely available.[6]

Molecular Testing

Traditional, or qualitative, PCR allows for detection of specific gene mutations or fusions via enzymatic replication of deoxyribonucleid acid (DNA) that is subsequently analyzed by methods such as gel or capillary electrophoresis. Qualitative PCR alerts only to the presence or absence of a target mutation, whereas quantitative real-time PCR specifies the amount of the target is present in a sample by measuring PCR amplification as it occurs. Digital PCR (dPCR) digitizes a bulk PCR mix into thousands of nanoliter-sized microreactions that can be examined independently using statistical software to determine the quantity of the target DNA with increasingly superior accuracy (10^{-4}; one mutation in 10,000 normal cells).[6] PCR turnaround time is generally 3 to 5 days.[15]

Sanger sequencing allows for detailed analysis of PCR fragments to detect small variations (<1 kb) by incorporation of fluorescently labeled dideoxynucleotides during DNA replication that are subsequently detected by electrophoresis.[6] It has the advantage of a relatively quick turnaround time but is limited by its high cost, labor intensity, limited analytical sensitivity (10^{-1}; abnormality must be present in at least 20% of cells), and requirement for expert interpretation in the cases of complex or unusual mutations.[16–18] Sanger sequencing is used for detecting mutations within a single exon such as CEBPA and is helpful in confirming PCR screening results, identifying potential germline variants, detecting specific base substitutions missed by PCR, or distinguishing between select benign versus pathogenic mutations that result similarly in PCR-based assays.[19]

NGS allows for the simultaneous evaluation of multiple genes with high sensitivity via analysis millions to billions of sequencing reactions run in parallel. NGS can be used to detect both small and large molecular abnormalities including single nucleotide variants, small insertions/deletions (indels) and depending on the design, may also be able to identify copy number alterations, gene fusions or chromosomal translocations, gene expression, and DNA methylation. It can assess multiple genes simultaneously (targeted gene panels; the most common NGS method in clinical laboratories), multiple genomic regions simultaneously (whole-exome sequencing), the full genome (whole genome sequencing [WGS]), or the whole transcriptome (whole-transcriptome sequencing). NGS is a semiquantitative method, expressing the proportion of a sample affected by a given mutation as the variant allele frequency (VAF) with typical analytical sensitivities of 2% to 5%.[6] NGS is limited by high cost, labor intensity, and interlaboratory differences in VAF measurement, assessment of pathogenicity of variants, and determination of germline versus somatic status of a mutation. Professional society guidelines are available to facilitate standardization of NGS result reporting.[20] Turnaround time is typically 5 to 14 days.[15]

Select molecular and cytogenetic methods are useful in monitoring minimal residual disease (MRD) following initial therapy in MDS and other myeloid malignancies. The least sensitive method available is FISH, with an analytical sensitivity of 10^{-2} to detect previously identified translocations such as RUNX1::RUNX1T1.[6] Quantitative PCR can be used to detect known molecular abnormalities with higher analytical sensitivities of 10^{-4} to 10^{-5}. dPCR remains exploratory in MRD monitoring, and the use of NGS for this purpose is limited by undefined VAF thresholds for residual disease among different mutations, lack of interlaboratory standardization of MRD monitoring techniques, and the challenge of distinguishing residual disease from premalignant clonal hematopoiesis (CH).[15]

The selection of given technology for molecular testing is based on a variety of factors including the type and number of molecular abnormalities tested, goal of testing (ie, diagnosis vs disease monitoring), cost of testing, time constraints, available labor and supplies in a clinical laboratory, and the availability of expert pathologists to interpret specific findings. Various techniques are best used in tandem, such as maximizing the sensitivity or PCR- or NGS-based assays while using the breadth of mutations detectable by Sanger sequencing. For example, in one case of a patient with AML with biallelic *CEBPA* mutation, the patient's somatic *CEBPA* mutation c.175 G greater than T was detected by NGS at a VAF of 6.6% missed by Sanger sequencing; however, Sanger sequencing and not NGS detected the patient's germline c.442 G > T mutation despite a VAF of 68%.[21]

GENE MUTATIONS IN MYELODYSPLASTIC SYNDROME

Owing to rapid advances in sequencing technology, dozens of driver mutations have been associated with MDS over the past decade, with 30 to 50 genes covered on a typical NGS panel.[22,23] Approximately 80% to 90% of MDS patients have at least one gene mutation, with most patients harboring two or three mutations at the time of diagnosis.[22–26] Broadly, a larger number of driver mutations are associated with poorer survival.[25–29] Gene mutations associated with MDS are grouped into functional classes in the literature based on their effects on DNA methylation, chromatin and histone modification, ribonucleic acid (RNA) splicing, the cohesin complex, transcription regulation, cytokine receptors/tyrosine kinases, the rat sarcoma (RAS) pathway, DNA repair, the cell cycle, and other signaling pathways (**Table 1**).[22,24–26] Mutations affecting DNA methylation and RNA splicing tend to occur early in disease progression, whereas mutations affecting chromatin modification and cellular signaling pathways tend to occur later.[22,28,30]

Among these pathways, mutations affecting splicing (*SF3B1*, *U2AF1*, *SRSF2*), DNA methylation (*DMNT3A*, *TET2*), and chromatin modification (*ASXL1*) are the most common in MDS (ie, > 10% of patients).[23–28,31,32] Some studies also document a high frequency of *TP53*[32] (tumor suppressor) and *RUNX1*[24,25,28] (transcription factor) mutations. Interestingly, there seem to be regional or ethnic differences in the prevalence

Table 1
Gene mutations associated with myelodysplastic syndrome

Functional Class	Genes
RNA splicing	*LUC7L2, PRPF8, SF1, **SF3B1**, **SRSF2**, **U2AF1**, U2AF2, ZRSR2*
DNA methylation	***DNMT3A**, IDH1, IDH2, **TET2**, WT1*
Chromatin and histone modification	***ASXL1**, ARID2, ATRX, EED, EZH2, JARID2, KDM6A, KMT2, SUZ12*
Cohesin complex	*RAD21, SMC1a, SMC3, STAG2*
Transcription regulation	*BCOR, BCORL1, CEBPA, CUX1, ETV6, GATA1, GATA2, IRF1, NCOR2, PHF6, **RUNX1***
Cytokine receptors/tyrosine kinases	*CALR, CSF3R, FLT3, JAK2, KIT, MPL*
RAS signaling	*CBL, KRAS, NF1, NRAS, PTPN11*
DNA repair	*ATM, BRCC3, FANCL*
Cell cycle	*CKDN2A, **TP53***
Other signaling	*DDX41, FBXW, GNAS, NOTCH1, PTEN, SETBP1*

Note: **Bolded** genes are those that are typically found in > 10% of MDS patients.

of certain mutations. For example, *SF3B1* mutations were found consistently less often in three Chinese studies[23,28,32] compared with European[25,26] and Indian studies.[27] In one Chinese study by Xu and colleagues, additional mutations affecting RNA splicing (*SRSF2*, *U2AF1*, *ZRSR2*) were found at lower frequencies as well compared with European studies.[28]

There is a significant overlap among driver mutations associated with MDS, AML, and premalignant CH, reflecting the process by which mutations accumulate over time by positive selection in the evolution of CH to MDS to AML from an initial clone.[30,33–36] CH is discussed in greater depth elsewhere in this review series, but briefly, it encompasses CH of indeterminate potential in which there exist MDS-associated gene mutations in the absence of cytopenias, as well as CH of uncertain significance (CCUS), in which there exist MDS-associated gene mutations and cytopenias without morphologic dysplasia. Recent research demonstrated that pathogenic mutations are acquired in a stepwise fashion in the progression from CH to MDS to AML with parallel progression in morphologic dysplasia, blast count, and MFC abnormalities. In this way, driver mutations are accumulated in a fashion that provides a survival advantage to the mutant hematopoietic stem cell precursor despite the downstream consequences of ineffective hematopoiesis.[30] Co-occurrence of driver mutations is not always random, as certain mutations co-occur more frequently, whereas others never co-occur, suggesting functional interactions among different driver mutations leading to positive or negative selection in genomic evolution.[4] Below, mutations are discussed by functional class. See **Table 2** for a summary of mutations by their prognostic impact.

Splicing Factors

Mutations affecting the spliceosome affect more than half of MDS patients.[37] Among them, mutations in *SF3B1*, *SRSF2*, *U2AF1*, and *ZRSR2* are the most common, leading to errors in pre-mRNA (messenger RNA) splicing with downstream deleterious effects on protein synthesis and mitochondrial function.[38] These mutations tend to occur early in MDS evolution and influence the development of cooperating mutations in clonal expansion.[22] Splicing factor mutations occur in a mutually exclusive fashion, suggesting co-occurrence is not compatible with cellular survival.[4]

Table 2
Gene mutations with prognostic impact in myelodysplastic syndrome

Positive Impact		Negative Impact	
Gene	Affected outcome	Gene	Affected outcome
SF3B1	OS	ASXL1	OS
		DNMT3A	OS, PFS
		ETV6	OS
		RUNX1	OS, PFS
		SRSF2	OS, PFS
		IDH1/2	PFS
		TP53	OS, PFS
		U2AF1	OS

Note: Included in this table are mutations that have been associated with negative survival outcomes in at least two studies.

Abbreviations: OS, overall survival; PFS, progression-free survival.

MDS with mutated *SF3B1* is discussed extensively in a separate entry in this review series. Briefly, it is associated with a favorable prognosis and is now recognized as a distinct diagnostic entity in the WHO 5th edition classification as well as the recent ICC guidelines.[1,2] It is associated with the presence of greater than 5% ring sidero-blasts,[22,24] which is proposed to be due to effects on genes involved in mitochondrial iron transportation, leading to excess iron deposition surrounding the mitochondria.[39] Nonetheless, current diagnostic criteria recognize MDS with *SF3B1* mutation as a ho-mogenous entity regardless of the number of ring sideroblasts or dysplastic cellular lineages.[24] Clinically, MDS with mutated *SF3B1* is associated with isolated anemia, normal or elevated platelet count, single or multilineage dysplasia, and low percentage of bone marrow blasts.[22,26] Most driver mutations and CNAs are less likely to subse-quently develop in the presence of an *SF3B1* mutation, with the exception of *DNMT3A*, *TET2*, *JAK2*, and del(5q).[4,25] Last, although generally associated with a favorable prognosis, *SF3B1* mutations are found in most cases of *EVI1* (*MECOM*) rear-rangements, which are associated with poor survival outcomes.[40,41]

SRSF2 mutations are associated with inferior outcomes in some but not all studies, including shorter overall survival,[22,42] higher risk International Prognostic Scoring Sys-tem (IPSS) score,[27] and shorter progression-free survival.[28] They are associated with trisomy 8 as well as the development of other driver mutations with distinct clinical fea-tures.[22] *SRSF2* mutation with concurrent *TET2* mutations is associated with a single cytopenia (usually anemia), multilineage dysplasia, and fewer than 10% bone marrow blasts, whereas commonly co-occurring *ASXL1*, *RUNX1*, *IDH2*, or *EZH2* mutations are associated with two or more cytopenias, multilineage dysplasia, and blasts greater than 10%.[22,25]

Research on the prognostic impact of *U2AF1* is inconsistent, with some studies reporting no impact on survival,[25,42] and others associating these mutations with decreased overall survival[32,43] and a higher risk IPSS score.[27] In one large study, *U2AF1* mutations were associated with co-occurrence of 20q deletion and chromo-some 7 abnormalities as well as a higher rate of transfusion-dependent anemia, multi-lineage dysplasia, and excess blasts.[22] *U2AF1* mutations are also associated with grade 2 to 3 marrow fibrosis,[43] and in Zhang and colleagues' recent study, they appeared in 40% of patients classified as MDS with fibrosis under the 5th edition WHO criteria.[24]

ZRSR2 mutations, though common, seem to have no impact on survival.[27,42] One European study found that the less common splicing factor mutation *PRPF8* is asso-ciated with poorer survival, though this finding is not consistently replicated.[25] Other splicing factor mutations such as those affecting *SF1* and *LUC7L2* are rarely observed in MDS and have not been clearly associated with survival outcomes.[4]

DNA Methylation

Mutations in a small number of genes affecting DNA methylation are implicated in the pathogenesis of MDS. The role of methylation pathways in MDS pathogenesis is sup-ported by the therapeutic efficacy of hypomethylating agents, azacitidine and decitabine.[44]

The gene *DNMT3A* encodes an enzyme involved in the de novo DNA methylation of cytosine.[4] Although often associated with a normal karyotype,[32] *DNMT3A* mutations are associated with poorer survival.[22,28,32,45] These mutations tend to co-occur with mutations in *BCOR*, *IDH1*, and *NPM1* but are mutually exclusive of *ASXL1* muta-tions.[22] Clinically, *DNMT3A* mutations are associated with a greater number and severity of cytopenias, excess blasts, and a greater rate of progression to AML.[22,45]

The genes *IDH1* and *IDH2* encode for isoforms of isocitrate dehydrogenase, a crit-ical enzyme involved in the citric acid cycle; when mutated, they instead catalyze the conversion of alpha-ketoglutarate into an oncometabolite that inhibits several enzymes involved in demethylation, including the product of *TET2*.[4] These mutations occur in around 10% of MDS patients[46] and are associated with poor outcomes including shorter overall survival[22] and higher risk IPSS score.[27] Interestingly, in one study, *IDH1/IDH2* mutations were associated with longer progression free survival.[28] Clinically, like *DNMT3A* mutations, *IDH1/IDH2* mutations are associated with multiple cytopenias, transfusion-dependence, excess blasts, and higher risk of leukemic progression.[22,26] These mutations are targeted by the therapeutic agents ivosidenib (*IDH1*) and enasidenib (*IDH2*) in cases of hypomethylating agent failure.[47]

   TET2 is involved in the early steps of DNA demethylation of cytosine.[4] Although it has been suggested that the mutation burden of *TET2* mutation may be negatively associated with survival,[48] the mere presence of *TET2* mutations does not seem to be associated with overall survival.[27,31] One study found *TET2* mutations to be associated with shorter progression-free survival, however.[28] Mutations in *WT1* have been associated with greater than 10% bone marrow blasts in two studies but have not been found to significantly correlate with overall survival.[24,26]

Chromatin Modification

Several genes mutated in MDS affect chromatin and histone modification, largely via impacts on the polycomb repressive complex 2 (*PRC2*), a large protein complex involved in the repression of genes involved in hematopoiesis.[4] The most important among these genes is *ASXL1*, which is associated with poorer overall survival in several studies.[23,25,27,31,32] *ASXL1* mutations occur in about 20% of MDS patients[25] and are associated with concurrent mutations in *SRSR2*, *RUNX1*, and *NRAS*.[22] Mutations in *ASXL1* are associated with faster progression to AML[32] and are also seen in chronic myelomonocytic leukemia and myeloproliferative neoplasms.[49,50] *EZH2* mutations, also related to chromatin modification, may be associated with poorer survival as well,[31] though this finding is not consistently replicated across studies.[28]

TP53 Mutation

Mutations in the *TP53* tumor suppressor gene are the most common in all human cancers.[51] In MDS specifically, biallelic *TP53* mutations are overwhelmingly associated with decreased overall survival,[22–25,27,28,31,32,46] including in patients who undergo allogeneic hematopoietic stem cell transplantation.[52,53] The vast majority of patients with biallelic *TP53* mutations exhibit complex karyotype,[22] though concurrent driver mutations are less likely to be found.[26,32] Clinically, *TP53* mutations are present in about half of cases of therapy-related MDS[54] and are associated with two or more cytopenias, transfusion-dependence, increased bone marrow blasts, faster rates of leukemic progression, and therapy resistance.[22,24,31] MDS with biallelic *TP53* mutation is discussed extensively in a separate article in this review series.

Other Mutations

Around 10% to 15% of MDS patients harbor mutations affecting the cohesin complex (eg, *STAG2*, *SMC1A*), which participates in the regulation of gene expression via large chromatin structures.[4] Similar to those affecting the spliceosome, mutations affecting the cohesin complex are typically mutually exclusive of each other.[55] One mechanism by which cohesin complex mutations contribute to MDS pathogenesis is accessibility to transcription factors such as *RUNX1* and *GATA2* by cohesin-deficient cells.[56] Cohesin complex mutations are found among both low- and high-risk MDS patients.[55]

   Acquisition of mutations affecting transcription factors is hypothesized to play a role in the progression from MDS to AML as reflected by the generally inferior outcomes associated with mutations in this group.[30] The most notable among these mutations are those affecting *RUNX1*, which are associated with poorer overall survival[25,31,32] and shorter progression-free survival.[28] Clinically, *RUNX1* mutations are associated with severe thrombocytopenia, excess blasts, and a greater rate of leukemic transformation.[22,31] Other transcription factor mutations that have been associated with poor overall survival outcomes include *ETV6*[28,31] and *GATA1/GATA2*.[28] Mutations in *BCOR* are associated with greater than 10% bone marrow blasts but not necessarily with overall survival.[24]

Mutations in genes encoding for cytokine receptors and tyrosine kinases are associated with MDS. Among these, *FLT3* mutations have been described as "AML-like" in that they are associated with multiple cytopenias, transfusion dependency, excess blasts, a greater rate of leukemic evolution, and poor prognosis.[22] *JAK2* mutations in MDS have been associated with poor overall survival in one study[27] and are associated with MDS/MPN (myeloproliferative neoplasm) overlap and thrombocytosis.[22] Other mutations in this class include *KIT*, *MPL*, *CALR*, and *CSF3R*.[4]

Mutations affecting *RAS* signaling can be seen in MDS and are generally clinically unfavorable.[57] *KRAS* mutations are associated with poorer overall survival.[25,27,28] *NRAS* mutations are similarly associated with poorer overall survival,[27,28] as well as greater risk of transformation to AML, severe thrombocytopenia, and increased bone marrow blasts.[26,28,31]

A variety of other mutations are found in a small number of MDS patients and are not known to affect survival, including those affecting genes involved in other signaling pathways (eg, *GNAS*, *PTEN*), DNA repair (eg, *ATM*), and gene expression (eg, *SETBP1*).[27,58–60]

Special Circumstances

Select gene mutations are associated with relapse rates following allogeneic hematopoietic stem cell transplantation (HSCT). Similar to patients who do not undergo HSCT, *SF3B1* mutations are associated with favorable survival outcomes following HSCT.[22] The most commonly reported mutations associated with inferior survival following HSCT in MDS patients are *TP53*,[22,52,61,62] *U2AF1*,[22,61] and *RAS* pathway mutations,[61,62] with individual studies additionally identifying *ASXL1*, *RUNX1*, and *IDH2*.[52,61] In Yoshizato and colleagues' study, *RAS* pathway mutations were associated with inferior survival only when a reduced intensity conditioning regimen was used, whereas *TP53* mutations were associated with poor survival regardless of conditioning regimen.[53]

Recent research demonstrates that at least 10% of patients with MDS have an inherited disposition to myeloid malignancy.[63] Consideration should be made to the presence of germline mutations in all MDS patients, but particularly in younger patients who harbor mutations in genes associated with hereditary predisposition for myeloid malignancy such as *GATA2*, *PIGA*, *DDX41*, or *SBDS*.[62,64,65] This issue is particularly relevant when considering HSCT, as potential donors in the family may harbor similar germline mutations that could lead to the development of a donor-derived myeloid malignancy.[66]

Weinberg and Hasserjian highlight that although select mutations may rarely be associated with MDS, their presence in cytopenic patients undergoing evaluation should suggest consideration of alternative diagnoses.[37] For example, a cytopenic patient with a *BRAF* mutation should be evaluated for hairy cell leukemia,[67] whereas one with *STAT3* or *STAT5B* mutations should be evaluated for large granular lymphocytic leukemia, which may clinically mimic MDS but requires different treatment.[68] The presence of the *KIT* codon 816 mutation should prompt consideration of systemic mastocytosis.[37] Clinicians should also be aware that in the WHO-HAEM5, mutations in *NPM1* now automatically default to a diagnosis of AML regardless of blast percentage due to evidence that patients with CH, MDS, or MDS/MPN who acquire NPM1 mutations tend to progress rapidly to AML and may benefit from earlier AML-directed therapy. AML can be diagnosed with a blast count less than 20% in the presence of characteristic rearrangements in *KMT2A*, *MECOM*, and *NUP98* as well.[1]

Last, there are MDS patients in whom genetic mutations are never detected. Some of these patients harbor cytogenetic abnormalities, but there exists a unique group with no associated genetic abnormalities.[22] In a recent large study conducted across the European Union, these patients were characterized by younger age, isolated anemia, normal or reduced marrow cellularity adjusted for age, absence of ring sideroblasts, low percentage of bone marrow blasts, and favorable prognosis with or without HSCT.[22] Other investigators have argued that in the era of expansive gene panels, in patients with isolated cytopenias, no marrow dysplasia, and no detectable genetic abnormalities; other diagnoses should be favored above MDS, including metabolic deficiencies, drug or toxin exposure (eg, azathioprine, methotrexate, alcohol), autoimmune disease (eg, systemic lupus erythematosus, Felty syndrome), or infections (eg, human immunodeficiency virus).[37,64]

DISCUSSION

MDS is increasingly understood as a genetically defined heterogenous entity that encompasses a range of disease from those at risk of progression to AML and mortality in less than a year, to others who live with relatively indolent disease for a decade or more.[69] Although many driver mutations have been identified, the prognostic significance and functional roles of these mutations in MDS pathogenesis are not consistently clear, with the exception of one mutation consistently associated with favorable outcomes (*SF3B1*) and a handful of mutations generally reported to be deleterious to overall survival (*TP53*, *ASXL1*, *RUNX1*, *DNMT3A*, *KRAS*, *NRAS*).[4] Unfortunately, there remain disagreements on standardized methods for genetic testing and analysis of gene mutations in MDS as well as which mutations to prioritize in a revised prognostication score system. In addition, the clinical significance of certain variables in genetic testing such as VAF, mutation type, and mutation location remain unclear for many genes.[64]

Increasing availability, affordability, and standardization of NGS assays herald a new era of MDS care. On the horizon are WGS techniques that have already been shown to provide fast and accurate genomic profiling of AML and MDS, with greater diagnostic yield than conventional methods, especially in cases with high genetic complexity.[70,71] The feasibility of this approach has recently been demonstrated in pediatric oncology,[72] and this technology is expected to outperform current technology in the coming years.[69] Other innovative methods that may be used to replace conventional cytogenetics include mate pair sequencing and optical genome mapping, which provide whole-genome analyses that efficiently detect copy number abnormalities and structural abnormalities, including balanced rearrangements missed by CMAs.[6,7] With the increased recognition of the role of germline predisposition to myeloid malignancy, molecular profiling is expected to focus on both somatic and germline testing for all patients in the future. Taken together, these technological advances may pave the way for a world in which patients are diagnosed with mechanistically defined variants of MDS with refined prognostication and individualized treatment approaches in addition to efficient identification of candidacy for clinical trials using targeted agents.[69]

For the past decade, risk stratification in MDS diagnosis has been based on the Revised IPSS (IPSS-R) which is based on clinical factors such as hemoglobin level, platelet count, absolute neutrophil count, and percentage of bone marrow blasts in addition to select cytogenetic abnormalities.[73] A known weakness of the IPSS-R is the classification of certain patients as low risk, who nonetheless experience inferior clinical outcomes compared with other members of that risk group.[5,74] Several investigators have attempted to devise a new prognostication tool that incorporates genetic data.[22,27,28,75,76] In response, the International Working Group for Prognosis in MDS recently published the IPSS-Molecular (IPSS-M), which adds to the IPSS-R 16 prognostic genes and an additional feature representing the number of mutations from an additional pool of 15 genes. Scoring produces a number on a continuous index which provides prognostic information for estimated leukemia-free survival, risk of leukemic transformation, and overall survival.[77] The IPSS-M was subsequently validated in a sample of 1281 MDS patients, demonstrating an ability of the IPSS-M to further risk stratify patients based on genetic features who were previously assigned to the low-risk group based on clinical and cytogenetic factors alone.[78] Further validation in diverse clinical scenarios is required to establish general clinical utility of this tool.

As prognostication refines, opportunities for targeted therapy emerge. Hypomethylating agents remain the first-line therapies for most MDS patients, though many patients fail to respond to these agents or eventually experience disease progression despite them. For those patients, several targeted therapies are available (some in clinical trials only) based on the presence of certain clinical or genetic features such as ring sideroblasts (luspatercept), deletion 5q (lenalidomide), IDH1 (ivosidenib), IDH2 (enasidenib), FLT3 (quizartinib, sorafenib, midostaurin, gilteritinib), spliceosome mutations (H3B-8800), TP53 (eprenetapopt), among others.[4,47,78] Current experimental therapies for MDS as of 2022 are discussed thoroughly in a recent review by Bazinet and colleagues.[79]

Last, as highlighted by Maurya and Jiang in their respective studies, several characteristics of MDS including age of onset, risk group, and the type and frequency of genetic mutations and chromosomal abnormalities appear to vary by national origin and/or ethnic group.[27,80] For example, Jiang and colleagues found that MDS cases in East Asia demonstrated a two- to fourfold lower incidence and a 10-year younger age of onset compared with Western data. Their study additionally showed that East Asian MDS patients were more likely to be categorized as intermediate, high, or very high risk according to IPSS compared with Western patients.[80] Maurya and colleagues similarly found a lower median age of MDS diagnosis (55 years) in South Asian patients and proposed that these differences may be due to different genetic susceptibilities among ethnic groups, dietary differences, or occupational and environmental toxic exposures.[27] Investigation into the nature of these differences may lead to greater understanding of MDS biology as a whole and elucidate ways to prevent development of MDS at younger ages in certain regions where there may be greater hereditary or environmental risk.

SUMMARY

The importance of gene mutations in the pathogenesis of MDS has become clearer in recent years following the widespread adaptation of NGS. Mutations affecting splicing and chromatin modification are the most common in MDS. Though there is some inconsistency in the literature regarding the effect on survival of many mutations, the beneficial effect of SF3B1 mutation and the deleterious effect of balletic TP53 mutation are well-documented. Other mutations that are reported to negatively impact overall survival include *ASXL1*, *RUNX1*, *DNMT3A*, and *RAS* pathway mutations. Updated WHO-HAEM5 and ICC guidelines as well as the new IPSS-M incorporate molecular data into the diagnosis and prognostication of MDS compared with older tools that were based on clinical or cytogenetic features only. With WGS methods predicted to become the new standard of genetic evaluation in the future, it is likely that MDS diagnosis and management will become increasingly personalized based on an individual's clinical and genomic profile.

CLINICS CARE POINTS

- Gene mutations that affect DNA methylation, chromatin modification, RNA splicing, the cohesin complex, transcription, cytokine receptors/tyrosine kinases, the RAS pathway, DNA repair, the cell cycle, and other signaling pathways are implicated in myelodysplastic syndrome (MDS) pathogenesis and often have prognostic, clinical, and therapeutic implications.

- Massively parallel gene sequencing technologies have facilitated a new era of MDS diagnosis and treatment that is characterized by genetically informed prognostication and targeted therapies.

- Updated World Health Organization-HAEM5 and International Consensus Classification schemes for 2022 highlight genetically defined entities within MDS, including MDS with *SF3B1* mutation, which is associated with favorable prognosis, and MDS with biallelic *TP53* mutation, which is associated with poor prognosis.

- Specific gene mutations and a variable reflecting the number of total gene mutations are incorporated into the updated International Prognostic Scoring System-Molecular, which provides a number on a continuous index for estimated leukemia-free survival, risk of leukemic transformation, and overall survival.

FUNDING AND CONFLICTS OF INTEREST

The authors report no relevant conflicts of interest, financial or otherwise.

REFERENCES

1. Khoury JD, Solary E, Abla O, et al. The 5th edition of the world Health organization classification of haematolymphoid tumours: myeloid and histiocytic/dendritic neoplasms. Leukemia 2022;36(7):1703–19.
2. Arber DA, Orazi A, Hasserjian RP, et al. International Consensus classification of myeloid neoplasms and acute leukemias: integrating morphologic, clinical, and genomic data. Blood 2022;140(11):1200–28.
3. Sun LM, Lin CL, Lin MC, et al. Radiotherapy- and chemotherapy-induced myelodysplasia syndrome: a nationwide population-based nested case-control study. Medicine (Baltim) 2015;94(17):e737.
4. Ogawa S. Genetics of MDS. Blood 2019;133(10):1049–59.
5. Zeidan AM, Shallis RM, Wang R, et al. Epidemiology of myelodysplastic syndromes: why characterizing the beast is a prerequisite to taming it. Blood Rev 2019;34:1–15.
6. Duncavage EJ, Bagg A, Hasserjian RP, et al. Genomic profiling for clinical decision making in myeloid neoplasms and acute leukemia. Blood 2022;140(21):2228–47.
7. Akkari YMN, Baughn LB, Dubuc AM, et al. Guiding the global evolution of cytogenetic testing for hematologic malignancies. Blood 2022;139(15):2273–84.

8. Mitelman F. Catalogue of chromosome aberrations in cancer. Cytogenet Cell Genet 1983;36(1–2):1–515.

9. Moorman AV, Harrison CJ, Buck GA, et al. Karyotype is an independent prognostic factor in adult acute lymphoblastic leukemia (ALL): analysis of cytogenetic data from patients treated on the Medical Research Council (MRC) UKALLXII/ Eastern Cooperative Oncology Group (ECOG) 2993 trial. Blood 2007;109(8): 3189–97.

10. Mallo M, Arenillas L, Espinet B, et al. Fluorescence in situ hybridization improves the detection of 5q31 deletion in myelodysplastic syndromes without cytogenetic evidence of 5q. Haematologica 2008;93(7):1001–8.

11. Coleman JF, Theil KS, Tubbs RR, et al. Diagnostic yield of bone marrow and peripheral blood FISH panel testing in clinically suspected myelodysplastic syndromes and/or acute myeloid leukemia: a prospective analysis of 433 cases. Am J Clin Pathol 2011;135(6):915–20.

12. Seegmiller AC, Wasserman A, Kim AS, et al. Limited utility of fluorescence in situ hybridization for common abnormalities of myelodysplastic syndrome at first presentation and follow-up of myeloid neoplasms. Leuk Lymphoma 2014;55(3): 601–5.

13. Rack KA, van den Berg E, Haferlach C, et al. European recommendations and quality assurance for cytogenomic analysis of haematological neoplasms: reponse to the comments from the Francophone Group of Hematological Cytogenetics (GFCH). Leukemia 2020;34(8):2262–4.

14. Maciejewski JP, Tiu RV, O'Keefe C. Application of array-based whole genome scanning technologies as a cytogenetic tool in haematological malignancies. Br J Haematol 2009;146(5):479–88.

15. Dohner H, Wei AH, Appelbaum FR, et al. Diagnosis and management of AML in adults: 2022 recommendations from an international expert panel on behalf of the ELN. Blood 2022;140(12):1345–77.

16. Behdad A, Weigelin HC, Elenitoba-Johnson KS, et al. A clinical grade sequencing-based assay for CEBPA mutation testing: report of a large series of myeloid neoplasms. J Mol Diagn 2015;17(1):76–84.

17. Mendoza H, Podoltsev NA, Siddon AJ. Laboratory evaluation and prognostication among adults and children with CEBPA-mutant acute myeloid leukemia. Int J Lab Hematol 2021;43(Suppl 1):86–95.

18. Smith TA, Whelan J, Parry PJ. Detection of single-base mutations in a mixed population of cells: a comparison of SSCP and direct sequencing. Genet Anal Tech Appl 1992;9(5–6):143–5.

19. Ahn JY, Seo K, Weinberg O, et al. A comparison of two methods for screening CEBPA mutations in patients with acute myeloid leukemia. J Mol Diagn 2009; 11(4):319–23.

20. Li MM, Datto M, Duncavage EJ, et al. Standards and guidelines for the interpretation and reporting of sequence variants in cancer: a joint Consensus recommendation of the association for molecular pathology, American society of clinical oncology, and college of American pathologists. J Mol Diagn 2017;19(1):4–23.

21. Mendoza H, Chen PH, Pine AB, et al. A case of acute myeloid leukemia with unusual germline CEBPA mutation: lessons learned about mutation detection, location, and penetrance. Leuk Lymphoma 2021;62(5):1251–4.

22. Bersanelli M, Travaglino E, Meggendorfer M, et al. Classification and personalized prognostic assessment on the basis of clinical and genomic features in myelodysplastic syndromes. J Clin Oncol 2021;39(11):1223–33.

23. Yu J, Li Y, Li T, et al. Gene mutational analysis by NGS and its clinical significance in patients with myelodysplastic syndrome and acute myeloid leukemia. Exp Hematol Oncol 2020;9:2.

24. Zhang Y, Wu J, Qin T, et al. Comparison of the revised 4th (2016) and 5th (2022) editions of the World Health Organization classification of myelodysplastic neoplasms. Leukemia 2022;36(12):2875–82.

25. Haferlach T, Nagata Y, Grossmann V, et al. Landscape of genetic lesions in 944 patients with myelodysplastic syndromes. Leukemia 2014;28(2):241–7.

26. Papaemmanuil E, Gerstung M, Malcovati L, et al. Clinical and biological implications of driver mutations in myelodysplastic syndromes. Blood 21 2013;122(22): 3616–27, quiz 3699.

27. Maurya N, Mohanty P, Dhangar S, et al. Comprehensive analysis of genetic factors predicting overall survival in Myelodysplastic syndromes. Sci Rep 2022; 12(1):5925.

28. Xu Y, Li Y, Xu Q, et al. Implications of mutational spectrum in myelodysplastic syndromes based on targeted next-generation sequencing. Oncotarget 2017;8(47): 82475–90.

29. Xu L, Gu ZH, Li Y, et al. Genomic landscape of CD34+ hematopoietic cells in myelodysplastic syndrome and gene mutation profiles as prognostic markers. Proc Natl Acad Sci U S A 2014;111(23):8589–94.

30. Gao L, Hyter S, Zhang D, et al. Morphologic, immunophenotypic, and molecular genetic comparison study in patients with clonal cytopenia of undetermined significance, myelodysplastic syndrome, and acute myeloid leukemia with myelodysplasia-related changes: a single institution experience. Int J Lab Hematol 2022;44(4):738–49.

31. Bejar R, Stevenson K, Abdel-Wahab O, et al. Clinical effect of point mutations in myelodysplastic syndromes. N Engl J Med 2011;364(26):2496–506.

32. Wu K, Nie B, Li L, et al. Bioinformatics analysis of high frequency mutations in myelodysplastic syndrome-related patients. Ann Transl Med 2021;9(19):1491.

33. Walter MJ, Shen D, Ding L, et al. Clonal architecture of secondary acute myeloid leukemia. N Engl J Med 2012;366(12):1090–8.

34. Malcovati L, Galli A, Travaglino E, et al. Clinical significance of somatic mutation in unexplained blood cytopenia. Blood 2017;129(25):3371–8.

35. Steensma DP. The clinical challenge of idiopathic cytopenias of undetermined significance (ICUS) and clonal cytopenias of undetermined significance (CCUS). Curr Hematol Malig Rep 2019;14(6):536–42.

36. Valent P, Orazi A, Steensma DP, et al. Proposed minimal diagnostic criteria for myelodysplastic syndromes (MDS) and potential pre-MDS conditions. Oncotarget 2017;8(43):73483–500.

37. Weinberg OK, Hasserjian RP. The current approach to the diagnosis of myelodysplastic syndromes(☆). Semin Hematol 2019;56(1):15–21.

38. Pellagatti A, Armstrong RN, Steeples V, et al. Impact of spliceosome mutations on RNA splicing in myelodysplasia: dysregulated genes/pathways and clinical associations. Blood 2018;132(12):1225–40.

39. Mupo A, Seiler M, Sathiaseelan V, et al. Hemopoietic-specific Sf3b1-K700E knock-in mice display the splicing defect seen in human MDS but develop anemia without ring sideroblasts. Leukemia 2017;31(3):720–7.

40. Lavallee VP, Gendron P, Lemieux S, et al. EVI1-rearranged acute myeloid leukemias are characterized by distinct molecular alterations. Blood 2015;125(1): 140–3.

41. Shiozawa Y, Malcovati L, Galli A, et al. Gene expression and risk of leukemic transformation in myelodysplasia. Blood 2017;130(24):2642–53.
42. Thol F, Kade S, Schlarmann C, et al. Frequency and prognostic impact of mutations in SRSF2, U2AF1, and ZRSR2 in patients with myelodysplastic syndromes. Blood 2012;119(15):3578–84.
43. Li B, Liu J, Jia Y, et al. Clinical features and biological implications of different U2AF1 mutation types in myelodysplastic syndromes. Genes Chromosomes Cancer 2018;57(2):80–8.
44. Yun S, Vincelette ND, Abraham I, et al. Targeting epigenetic pathways in acute myeloid leukemia and myelodysplastic syndrome: a systematic review of hypomethylating agents trials. Clin Epigenetics 2016;8:68.
45. Walter MJ, Ding L, Shen D, et al. Recurrent DNMT3A mutations in patients with myelodysplastic syndromes. Leukemia 2011;25(7):1153–8.
46. Hellstrom-Lindberg E, Tobiasson M, Greenberg P. Myelodysplastic syndromes: moving towards personalized management. Haematologica 2020;105(7): 1765–79.
47. Montalban-Bravo G, Garcia-Manero G, Jabbour E. Therapeutic choices after hypomethylating agent resistance for myelodysplastic syndromes. Curr Opin Hematol 2018;25(2):146–53.
48. Jiang L, Luo Y, Zhu S, et al. Mutation status and burden can improve prognostic prediction of patients with lower-risk myelodysplastic syndromes. Cancer Sci 2020;111(2):580–91.
49. Carbuccia N, Murati A, Trouplin V, et al. Mutations of ASXL1 gene in myeloproliferative neoplasms. Leukemia 2009;23(11):2183–6.
50. Gelsi-Boyer V, Trouplin V, Adelaide J, et al. Mutations of polycomb-associated gene ASXL1 in myelodysplastic syndromes and chronic myelomonocytic leukaemia. Br J Haematol 2009;145(6):788–800.
51. Boutelle AM, Attardi LD. p53 and tumor suppression: it takes a network. Trends Cell Biol 2021;31(4):298–310.
52. Della Porta MG, Galli A, Bacigalupo A, et al. Clinical effects of driver somatic mutations on the outcomes of patients with myelodysplastic syndromes treated with allogeneic hematopoietic stem-cell transplantation. J Clin Oncol 2016;34(30): 3627–37.
53. Yoshizato T, Nannya Y, Atsuta Y, et al. Genetic abnormalities in myelodysplasia and secondary acute myeloid leukemia: impact on outcome of stem cell transplantation. Blood 2017;129(17):2347–58.
54. Wong TN, Ramsingh G, Young AL, et al. Role of TP53 mutations in the origin and evolution of therapy-related acute myeloid leukaemia. Nature 2015;518(7540): 552–5.
55. Thota S, Viny AD, Makishima H, et al. Genetic alterations of the cohesin complex genes in myeloid malignancies. Blood 2014;124(11):1790–8.
56. Noutsou M, Li J, Ling J, et al. The cohesin complex is necessary for epidermal progenitor cell function through maintenance of self-renewal genes. Cell Rep 2017;20(13):3005–13.
57. Akram AM, Chaudhary A, Kausar H, et al. Analysis of RAS gene mutations in cytogenetically normal de novo acute myeloid leukemia patients reveals some novel alterations. Saudi J Biol Sci 2021;28(7):3735–40.
58. Morotti A, Panuzzo C, Crivellaro S, et al. The role of PTEN in myeloid malignancies. Hematol Rep 2015;7(4):5844.
59. Fragoso R, Barata JT. PTEN and leukemia stem cells. Adv Biol Regul 2014; 56:22–9.

60. Ribeiro HL Jr, Oliveira RT, Maia AR, et al. ATM polymorphism is associated with low risk myelodysplastic syndrome. DNA Repair 2013;12(2):87–9.
61. Heuser M, Gabdoulline R, Loffeld P, et al. Individual outcome prediction for myelodysplastic syndrome (MDS) and secondary acute myeloid leukemia from MDS after allogeneic hematopoietic cell transplantation. Ann Hematol 2017;96(8):1361–72.
62. Lindsley RC, Saber W, Mar BG, et al. Prognostic mutations in myelodysplastic syndrome after stem-cell transplantation. N Engl J Med 2017;376(6):536–47.
63. Kennedy AL, Shimamura A. Genetic predisposition to MDS: clinical features and clonal evolution. Blood 2019;133(10):1071–85.
64. Voso MT, Gurnari C. Have we reached a molecular era in myelodysplastic syndromes? Hematology Am Soc Hematol Educ Program 2021;2021(1):418–27.
65. Chlon TM, Stepanchick E, Hershberger CE, et al. Germline DDX41 mutations cause ineffective hematopoiesis and myelodysplasia. Cell Stem Cell 4 2021; 28(11):1966–1981 e6.
66. Feurstein S, Trottier AM, Estrada-Merly N, et al. Germ line predisposition variants occur in myelodysplastic syndrome patients of all ages. Blood 2022;140(24):2533–48.
67. Tiacci E, Trifonov V, Schiavoni G, et al. BRAF mutations in hairy-cell leukemia. N Engl J Med 2011;364(24):2305–15.
68. Rajala HL, Eldfors S, Kuusanmaki H, et al. Discovery of somatic STAT5b mutations in large granular lymphocytic leukemia. Blood 2013;121(22):4541–50.
69. Cazzola M. Risk stratifying MDS in the time of precision medicine. Hematology Am Soc Hematol Educ Program 2022;2022(1):375–81.
70. Duncavage EJ, Schroeder MC, O'Laughlin M, et al. Genome sequencing as an alternative to cytogenetic analysis in myeloid cancers. N Engl J Med 2021; 384(10):924–35.
71. Haferlach T, Hutter S, Meggendorfer M. Genome sequencing in myeloid cancers. N Engl J Med 2021;384(25):e106.
72. Shukla N, Levine MF, Gundem G, et al. Feasibility of whole genome and transcriptome profiling in pediatric and young adult cancers. Nat Commun 2022;13(1):2485.
73. Greenberg PL, Tuechler H, Schanz J, et al. Revised international prognostic scoring system for myelodysplastic syndromes. Blood 20 2012;120(12):2454–65.
74. DeZern AE. Lower risk but high risk. Hematology Am Soc Hematol Educ Program 2021;2021(1):428–34.
75. Nazha A, Al-Issa K, Hamilton BK, et al. Adding molecular data to prognostic models can improve predictive power in treated patients with myelodysplastic syndromes. Leukemia 2017;31(12):2848–50.
76. Nazha A, Komrokji R, Meggendorfer M, et al. Personalized prediction model to risk stratify patients with myelodysplastic syndromes. J Clin Oncol 20 2021; 39(33):3737–46.
77. Bernard E, Tuechler H, Greenberg PL, et al. Molecular international pognostic scoring system for myelodyplastic syndromes. NEJM Evid 2022;1(7). https:// doi.org/10.1056/EVIDoa2200008.
78. Kewan T, Bahaj W, Durmaz A, et al. Validation of the molecular international prognostic scoring system in patients with myelodysplastic syndromes. Blood 2023. https://doi.org/10.1182/blood.2022018896.
79. Bazinet A, Bravo GM. New approaches to myelodysplastic syndrome treatment. Curr Treat Options Oncol 2022;23(5):668–87.
80. Jiang Y, Eveillard JR, Couturier MA, et al. Asian population is more prone to develop high-risk myelodysplastic syndrome, concordantly with their propensity to exhibit high-risk cytogenetic aberrations. Cancers 2021;13(3). https://doi.org/ 10.3390/cancers13030481.

Premalignant Clonal Hematopoiesis (Clonal Hematopoiesis of Indeterminate Potential and Clonal Cytopenia of Undetermined Significance)

Kelly E. Craven, MD, PhD[a], Mark D. Ewalt, MD[a],*

KEYWORDS

- Clonal hematopoiesis • Clonal hematopoiesis of indeterminate potential
- Clonal cytopenia of undetermined significance
- Paroxysmal nocturnal hemoglobinuria • VEXAS syndrome
- Therapy-related clonal hematopoiesis

KEY POINTS

- Clonal hematopoiesis (CH) is the presence of somatic alterations in the peripheral blood of individuals without evidence of a hematologic malignancy.
- When alterations are present in known hematologic-malignancy-related genes, the more specific term clonal hematopoiesis of indeterminate potential (CHIP) is used.
- CH and CHIP are often used somewhat interchangeably. Incidental somatic mutations, patients may present with unexplained cytopenia(s) without somatic mutations and are referred to as having idiopathic cytopenia of undetermined significance (ICUS).
- Patients with both unexplained cytopenia(s) and somatic mutations are designated as having clonal cytopenia of undetermined significance (CCUS).
- It is estimated that only 35% to 50% of ICUS patients meet the criteria for CCUS, though individuals with multiple cytopenias or mild dysplasia below the threshold required to diagnose myelodysplastic syndrome (MDS) are more likely to have mutations.
- When CCUS occurs alongside significant dysplasia, increased blasts, or MDS-defining genetic alterations, it is then considered MDS.

[a] Department of Pathology and Laboratory Medicine, Memorial Sloan Kettering Cancer Center, 1275 York Avenue, Box 36, New York, NY 10065, USA
* Corresponding author.
E-mail address: ewaltm@mskcc.org

Clin Lab Med 43 (2023) 565–576
https://doi.org/10.1016/j.cll.2023.06.001
0272-2712/23/© 2023 Elsevier Inc. All rights reserved.

labmed.theclinics.com

INTRODUCTION

Clonal hematopoiesis (CH) is the presence of somatic alterations in the peripheral blood of individuals without evidence of a hematologic malignancy.[1–4] When these alterations are present in known hematologic-malignancy-related genes and occur at a variant allele fraction (VAF) of at least 2% (4% in X-linked genes), the more specific term clonal hematopoiesis of indeterminate potential (CHIP) is used.[4–8] However, CH and CHIP are often used somewhat interchangeably. Aside from presenting with incidental somatic mutations, patients may present with unexplained cytopenia(s) (defined as anemia: hemoglobin < 13 g/dL in males or <12 g/dL in females; leukopenia: absolute neutrophil count <1.8 × 10^9/μL; or thrombocytopenia: platelets<150 × 10^9/μL) without somatic mutations and are referred to as having idiopathic cytopenia of undetermined significance (ICUS).[4,6,7] Patients with both unexplained cytopenia(s) and somatic mutations are designated as having clonal cytopenia of undetermined significance (CCUS)[6–9] (**Fig. 1**). It is estimated that only 35% to 50% of ICUS patients meet the criteria for CCUS,[2,10] though individuals with multiple cytopenias or mild dysplasia below the threshold required to diagnose myelodysplastic syndrome (MDS)[10] are more likely to have mutations.[2] When CCUS occurs alongside significant dysplasia, increased blasts, or MDS-defining genetic alterations, it is then considered MDS[6] (see **Fig. 1**).

CH was first broadly recognized in a series of population cohort studies that found the presence of somatic mutations in the peripheral blood.[1–3] To assess the relevance of these mutations to future hematologic malignancy, studies primarily focused on known cancer-associated[3] or hematologic malignancy-associated genes.[1–3] All studies showed that the frequency of individuals with mutations was higher in older age groups,[1–3] such that in one study, the frequency of individuals younger than

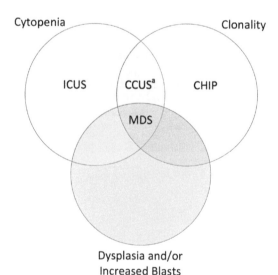

Fig. 1. Overlapping features of cytopenia, clonality, and morphologic findings in patients with idiopathic cytopenia of undetermined significance (ICUS), clonal cytopenia of undetermined significance (CCUS), clonal hematopoiesis of indeterminate potential (CHIP), and myelodysplastic syndrome (MDS). [a]Patients with cytopenia and specific genetic alterations, including biallelic TP53 mutation, isolated del(5q), and SF3B1 mutation rarely show no morphologic dysplasia or increase in blasts and may still be classified as MDS.[6,7]

50 years of age with mutations associated with hematologic malignancy was 0.7% compared with 5.7% in individuals over 65 years.[1] This incidence increased up to 10.4% in individuals over 65 years as compared with 0.9% in individuals younger than 50 years when a larger group of mutations were considered.[1] More recent studies with highly sensitive sequencing techniques (VAF $\geq$ 0.01%) have shown that CH can be identified in even young adults suggesting that ongoing somatic mutation occurs in all progenitors but a fitness advantage is required to drive clonal expansion to the level of VAF greater than or equal to 2% that is diagnostic for CHIP.[11–13]

CLINICAL IMPLICATIONS OF CLONAL HEMATOPOIESIS

Although many individuals with CH never go on to develop a hematologic malignancy,[10] several studies have shown that they are at markedly increased risk for blood cancer compared with individuals without CH, with hazard ratios (HRs) ranging from 11.1 (95% confidence interval (CI) 3.9–32.6)[2] to 12.9 (95% CI 5.8–28.7)[1] (**Fig. 2**). In those with high ($\geq$10%) VAF, the risk of progression to hematopoietic neoplasm was even more marked with a HR of 49 (95% CI 21–120).[2] However, among patients with CHIP, the absolute risk of conversion to hematologic cancer is quite small at only 0.5% to 1% per year.[1,2] Individuals with CCUS are at an even higher risk of developing a myeloid neoplasm with a HR of 13.9 (95% CI 5.4–35.91) with an 82% probability of progression to myeloid neoplasm at 5 years.[14] The presence of a high ($\geq$10%) VAF had an 86% positive predictive value (PPV) for a myeloid neoplasm, whereas the presence of 2 or more mutations (VAF $\geq$2%, but not otherwise specified) had a PPV of 88% for myeloid neoplasm.[14]

Potentially more significant than the risk of hematologic malignancy in CHIP is the risk of cardiovascular disease (CAD) (HR 1.9–2) and ischemic stroke (HR 2.6).[2,15] These sequelae may account for the finding that individuals with CH have an increased risk for death (HR 1.4),[1,2] which cannot be explained by the development of hematologic cancers alone.[2] The mechanism behind the increased cardiovascular event risk is not fully understood; however, specific genes have been shown to confer risk including *DNMT3A*, *TET2*, *ASXL1*, and *JAK2*, with *JAK2* conferring the greatest risk with a 12 fold increase, compared with a 2 fold increase with the other genes.[15] Numerous studies have found that CH is associated with inflammatory conditions,

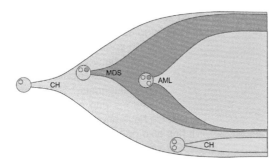

Fig. 2. Schematic of clonal evolution in hematopoietic cells with clonal hematopoiesis. In a single cell (*gray circle*), an initial mutation (*small blue circle*) is the founding event for CH. As the clone expands over time, it frequently acquires additional somatic hits which may be of uncertain malignant potential (*small green circle*) allowing the persistence of a more complex CH clone (*bottom*) or pathogenic (*small purple circle*) with progression to overt myelodysplastic syndrome (MDS) (*top*). With the acquisition of additional hits (*small orange circle*), the MDS clone progresses to acute myeloid leukemia (AML).

but it is unclear whether this association is causal. Pre-clinical model systems have suggested that CH could be causative, as some CH-related genes, such as *TET2*, can suppress inflammatory markers, and disruption of *TET2* by knockout or alteration has been shown to lead to increased tissue damage on inflammatory insult or increased atherosclerotic plaque size; however, the exact relationship of CH and inflammation is still under intense study.[15–18]

DISTINCTION FROM MYELODYSPLASTIC SYNDROME AND RISK OF PROGRESSION

By definition, CHIP lacks cytopenia, whereas this feature is a *sine qua non* of MDS, which makes the separation of these entities quite straightforward.[5–7] However, the distinction between CCUS and early MDS are more challenging. In addition to cytopenia, MDS requires the presence of significant ($\geq$10% of at least one hematopoietic lineage) morphologic dysplasia, increased blasts ($\geq$5% in bone marrow or $\geq$2% in peripheral blood), or the presence of an MDS-defining genetic alteration.[6,7] The most recent updates to the classification of hematologic malignancy, the International Consensus Classification of Myeloid Neoplasms and Acute Leukemias (ICC)[19] and the 5th edition of the World Health Organization (WHO) Classification of Haematolymphoid Tumours (WHO5)[6] detail these MDS-defining genetic alterations that may pose the greatest challenge in distinction from CCUS. Both classifications recognize 3 genetic subgroups that may not meet the above dysplasia threshold, but may still be diagnosed as MDS.[6,7] These groups are MDS with del(5q) (ICC)/MDS with low blasts and isolated 5q deletion (WHO5); MDS with mutated *TP53* (ICC)/MDS with biallelic *TP53* inactivation (WHO5); and MDS with mutated *SF3B1* (ICC)/MDS with low blasts and *SF3B1* mutation (WHO5).[6,7] In addition, the ICC requires a VAF greater than or equal to 10% for *SF3B1* mutations and requires 2 or more *TP53* mutations with VAF greater than or equal to 10%, or a single mutation with VAF greater than or equal to 10% along with complex karyotype or evidence of loss of heterozygosity or deletion of 17p in the region of the *TP53* gene for the mutated *SF3B1* and *TP53* categories, respectively.[7] At the time of this writing, the final version of WHO5 is not yet available; however, the initial article does not include an entity that corresponds to the ICC category of MDS not otherwise specified, which lacks dysplasia and is defined solely by MDS-defining cytogenetic abnormalities.[6,7]

One challenge of using morphologic dysplasia as a major criterion to differentiate CCUS from MDS is the inherent subjectivity involved in the evaluation of dysplasia, and the existence of many other non-neoplastic causes of dysplasia such as toxin, drug exposure, or nutritional deficiency.[4,20] In addition, minor morphologic abnormalities (ie, hypercellularity, hypocellularity, dysplasia, etc.) may be seen in patients with CHIP or CCUS; however, the extent of these findings is below the thresholds required to render a specific hematologic malignancy diagnosis.[4] This has raised the question of whether the presence of somatic mutations can or should be used in place of morphologic dysplasia; however, studies have shown that both CHIP and CCUS are far more frequent than MDS.[5,10] It has also been shown that while the overall survival (OS) of patients with CCUS (73.4% 5 year OS) is worse than those with non-clonal ICUS (89.4% 5 year OS), it is still superior to those with lower risk MDS (58.8% 5 year OS).[21] This suggests that purely broadening the diagnostic criteria to merge CCUS with low-grade MDS may lead to overdiagnosis. Therefore, others have focused on trying to identify specific genes or molecular parameters that may be useful to distinguish CCUS and MDS.

One approach to define molecular parameters predictive of progression is the use of mutation number or mutation VAF. An early study of 249 patients with ICUS performed with a 22 gene panel showed a higher mean mutation number in MDS patients (2.5) as compared with those with CCUS (1.3–1.5) and a trend to high-mutation VAF (33%) in MDS patients compared with those with CCUS and no morphologic dysplasia (23%).[10] A larger study of 873 patients with cytopenia using a 40 gene panel found that the presence of a somatic mutation had a PPV of 0.81 for the development of a myeloid neoplasm, and the presence of 2 or more had a PPV of 0.88.[14] This group also analyzed various VAF thresholds and found that a VAF of 8.7% had the best discriminatory ability between those who would subsequently develop a myeloid neoplasm with a PPV of 0.86.[14] In a subsequent study, this group replicated these findings with an increased risk for progression associated with the presence of a single mutation (HR 2.8) which markedly increased with 2 or more mutations (HR 7.9) or the presence of mutations with a VAF greater than or equal to 10% (HR 7.5).[22] Similarly, another study of 356 patients with CCUS found that the presence of greater than 1 somatic mutation had a marked increased risk of progression compared with a single mutation (HR 4.67).[23] In a study examining pre-leukemic samples of patients who progressed to AML in comparison with matched CH patients, pre-AML cases had significantly higher-mutation numbers per sample and 39% of these patients had mutations with a VAF greater than or equal to 10%, as compared with only 4% of controls who did not progress.[24] In addition to establishing the PPV of mutations and VAF, others have used the absence of mutations or abnormal karyotype (ICUS) to aid in ruling out a hematologic neoplasm. The absence of mutation in ICUS has a negative predictive value ranging from 84% to 95%[14,25] and the majority of cases of MDS show at least 1 mutation,[14,25–27] with a median of 9 coding mutations overall, across the exome.[27]

Aside from using the presence, number, and VAF of somatic mutations to define risk, many groups have examined the prognostic impact of mutations in specific genes. CHIP and CCUS show recurrent mutations in several key cellular signaling pathways (**Table 1**) including epigenetic regulation (ASXL1, DNMT3A, EZH2, IDH1/2, and TET2), RNA splicing (SF3B1, SRSF2, U2AF1, and ZRSR2), transcription factors (CUX1 and RUNX1), cell signaling (CBL, GNB1, JAK2, KRAS, and NRAS), and the DNA damage response (ATM, PPM1D, and TP53).[1–4,10,14,27–33] To identify which of these genes may be associated with a risk of progression to MDS, several groups have examined the incidence of recurrently mutated genes in CH (CHIP and CCUS) as compared with hematologic neoplasms. These studies have found that some of the most commonly mutated genes in CH including ASXL1, DNMT3A, JAK2, and TET2 are common both in individuals with CH as well as those with MDS or another hematologic malignancy, suggesting that these are earlier events in clonal evolution.[2,10,14,26,28,34] However, among these most commonly altered genes, mutations in DNMT3A and TET2 were seen at similar or higher incidence in CH suggesting a lower risk of progression.[9,26,34] Mutations in genes less frequently altered in CH, including CBL, CUX1, IDH1/2, NRAS, RUNX1, TP53, and splicing factor genes (SF3B1, SRSF2, U2AF1, and ZRSR2), have been found with a higher incidence in overt malignancy and/or are specifically associated with clonal progression and are therefore considered higher-risk mutations.[2,9,10,14,26–28,30,34,35]

Taken together these results suggest that risk factors for progression to MDS or a hematologic cancer are (1) the presence of 2 or more somatic mutations,[10,14,22,24,36] (2) the presence of somatic mutations with a higher VAF ($\geq$10%),[2,10,14,22,24,28,37] and (3) the presence of specific higher-risk mutations.[2,9,10,14,26–28,30,34,35] Patients harboring multiple risk factors also show increased risk. For example, one study showed that morphologic dysplasia was present when patients harbor 2 or more high-risk mutations (TP53 or SF3B1 plus at least one of DNMT3A, TET2, and/or

Table 1
Characteristics of frequently altered genes in clonal hematopoiesis

Pathway	Gene	Prevalence of Mutation in CH[a]	High Risk for Progression as Single Mutation
Cell Signaling	CBL	1–4%	Y
	GNB1	1–4%	Y
	JAK2	<1–10%	Y
	KRAS	<1–3%	Y
	NRAS	<1–2%	Y
DNA Damage Response	ATM	1–7%	Y
	PPM1D	<1 = 3%	Y
	TP53	<1–6%	Y
Epigenetics	ASXL1	3–16%	Y
	DNMT3A	8–50%	N
	EZH2	<1–4%	Y
	IDH1	<1–8%	Y
	IDH2	<1–5%	Y
	TET2	6–38%	?
Splicing	SF3B1	1–8%	Y
	SRSF2	1–21%	Y
	U2AF1	1–11%	Y
	ZRSR2	1–14%	Y
Transcription	CUX1	<1–3%	Y
	RUNX1	<1–6%	Y

Abbreviations: CH, Clonal Hematopoiesis; ?, the prognostic significance of *TET2* mutations is controversial.
    [a] Mutation prevalence based on data from several CH studies.[2,14,22,24,26,31,33–37]

ASXL1) with a VAF less than 20%, whereas for patients with lower-risk mutation patterns, dysplasia was not observed unless somatic mutation VAF greater than or equal to 30%.[22] The exact details of these complex interactions are an active area of continuing investigation.

THERAPY-RELATED CLONAL HEMATOPOIESIS

It has been recognized that myeloid neoplasms can result from previous exposure to cytotoxic therapy, such as alkylating agents, ionizing radiation, DNA topoisomerase II inhibitors, anti-metabolites, anti-tubulin agents, and PARP1 inhibitors.[6,19,38,39] As overt myeloid malignancy following therapy generally takes one to ten years to develop, and individuals with simultaneous CHIP (detected either before, during, or after cytotoxic therapy) have been shown to have an elevated risk of therapy-related myeloid neoplasm (t-MN),[32,40,41] therapy-related clonal hematopoiesis (t-CH), and clonal cytopenia (t-CC) have now become recognized premalignant entities.[19] Similar to non-therapy-related CH, the risk of progression to overt malignancy is also increased with more total mutations and larger clone size (higher VAF) in patients with therapy-related CH.[32]

Studies have shown that the mechanism of CH following therapy is not due to genome-wide DNA damage by the cytotoxic agent per se, but instead due to the selective expansion of existing low-level premalignant clones.[32,42] Consistent with this hypothesis is the finding that mutations present in pre-existing CH before treatment have been detected in the dominant clone at the transformation to overt t-MN.[32,42] In addition, patients who have received prior cancer-directed cytotoxic therapy are more likely to have CH than treatment-naive individuals, and a cumulative dose effect has been described with an increasing odds ratio of CH in those with increased exposure.[32] However, it is important to note that some individuals with t-CH after cancer-directed therapy will never progress to frank t-MN.[32] Another group found that only 30.3% of those with t-CC progressed to t-MN and the OS of patients with t-CC (OS 124.5 months) was significantly longer than those with t-MN (13–OS 16.3 months).[43]

Numerous groups have studied the altered genes in t-CH, particularly in patients with cancer, and have identified an increased incidence of mutations in DNA damage response genes CHEK2, PPM1D, and TP53, as compared with patients with CH unrelated to cytotoxic therapy,[32,40–46] which likely explains the increase in these mutations in patients with t-MN as compared with de novo disease.[42–45] Given that t-MNs may impact up to 25% of patients with cancer,[46] screening of this group for CH and other high-risk features (multiple somatic mutations, high VAF, and high-risk mutations) may identify those who deserve close follow-up.

UNIQUE CLONAL CYTOPENIA SYNDROMES

Although most cases of CCUS present with an isolated cytopenia and a somatic alteration that define clonality, there are rare syndromes in which t-CCs are associated with other specific clinical phenotypes. Although these syndromes are not considered malignant, their associated symptoms may require treatment and they all share an increased risk of progression to MDS. These syndromes include paroxysmal nocturnal hemoglobinuria (PNH) and vacuoles, E1 enzyme, X-linked, autoinflammatory, somatic (VEXAS) syndrome.

PNH is characterized by somatic mutations in the PIGA gene that lead to a defect in glycosylphosphatidylinositol (GPI) anchoring of proteins to the cell membrane and subsequent loss or marked deficiency of such proteins on the cell surface.[47,48] The loss of GPI-anchored proteins includes loss of the complement inhibitors CD55 (decay-accelerating factor) and CD59.[48,49] These factors usually inhibit complement and their loss leads to complement-mediated hemolysis that along with thrombosis, and potential for bone marrow failure are clinical hallmarks of the syndrome.[48,49] Although the somatic PIGA mutation is considered the cause of the patient's hemolytic phenotype, broad-based sequencing studies have shown more complex somatic mutation patterns including the presence of mutations in genes frequently associated with myeloid disease such as TET2, SUZ12, U2AF1, and JAK2.[48,50] These additional mutations may account for the risk of progression to frank MDS or AML in patients with PNH.[51,52]

The VEXAS syndrome was recently described through a genotype-driven analysis searching for recurrent alterations in an exome sequencing cohort of patients with undiagnosed recurrent fevers and/or systemic inflammation.[53] The initial study identified 25 male patients with somatic mutations affecting p.Met41 in the UBA1 gene which is found on the X chromosome and encodes the major E1-activating enzyme in the ubiquitination pathway.[53] Subsequent groups have expanded the spectrum of VEXAS-associated UBA1 mutations to include alterations affecting p.Ser56 and RNA splicing.[53–55] VEXAS-associated mutations disrupt the cytoplasmic isoform, Uba1b, causing defects in ubiquitin signaling which lead to the clinical features of VEXAS including markedly increased inflammation.[53,54,56] Clinically, the vast majority of patients (>95%) are male and all present with signs or symptoms of systemic inflammation including fever, multisystem inflammation (most commonly skin, lungs, and orbit).[53–55] Laboratory findings include macrocytic anemia and increased markers of inflammation while bone marrow morphologic assessment classically reveals the presence of cytoplasmic vacuoles in myeloid and erythroid precursors.[53–55,57,58] Similar to PNH, patients have an increased risk of subsequently developing a hematologic malignancy with progression to MDS being the most common and plasma cell neoplasms being frequently observed.[53,55,57,58] Also similar to PNH is the presence of frequent mutations in myeloid disease-associated genes, most commonly *DNMT3A*, which may also relate to the risk of transformation to overt myeloid malignancy.[53,58,59]

DISCUSSION

CH is a pre-malignant neoplastic process with significant implications for the health of affected patients. Given the marked increase in cardiovascular risk, increased attention should be paid to the management of comorbid conditions associated with heart disease. In addition, the recognition of t-MN arising both from t-CH and as the progression of underlying CH suggests that screening for CH before treatment of another malignancy may allow tailoring of therapy to prevent clonal progression that is accelerated with increasing cumulative cytotoxic exposure.

Although alterations in certain genes or a combination of genes have been associated with an increased risk of progression in CH, there is variability in the literature about specific combinations and thresholds that should prompt clinical action. Although additional studies are needed to refine these approaches, the application of artificial intelligence/machine learning technology may also allow for the development of a robust tool to distinguish those patients with the highest risk for progression. Such approaches have shown promise in MDS in which incorporation of molecular features provide better risk classification than the prior models.[60–63] By similarly identifying these high-risk patients with CH, clinical trials are designed to assess the efficacy of therapeutic intervention to prevent progression to overt hematologic neoplasia.

The past decade has seen an explosion in our understanding of the biology and clinical implications of CH. In the coming years, we hope to see progress in trials of clinical interventions which will mitigate the cardiovascular and neoplastic risks posed by the presence of this condition.

SUMMARY

CH is an aging-associated condition which was initially discovered from the analysis of somatic mutations in the peripheral blood of individuals from large population studies. In current classification systems, it is considered a premalignant condition that confers increased risk for hematologic malignancy (including those that are therapy related) as well as for CAD and death. As our knowledge of how the identified molecular alterations lead to perturbed signaling pathways continues to evolve, so will our ability to develop future interventions to avoid these consequences.

CLINICS CARE POINTS

- Premalignant CH is associated with an increased risk for the development of hematologic malignancy, particularly in patients with mutations in high-risk genes, those with high-mutation burden (VAF ≥10%), and those with mutations in multiple genes.

- Individuals with CH have an increased risk for CAD, which should prompt increased vigilance in the management of concomitant risk factors such as hypertension, high cholesterol, diabetes, obesity, and tobacco use.

- Therapy-related CH places individuals at an increased risk of therapy-related myeloid neoplasm following exposure to cytotoxic chemotherapy for another malignancy, and a cumulative dose effect has been described.
- The rare syndromes PNH and VEXAS syndrome are caused by somatic alterations and may be considered special cases of CH with specific clinical features and treatments. Like other CH cases, patients with these syndromes also have an increased risk of hematologic malignancy.

DISCLOSURE

The authors have nothing to disclose.

FUNDING

This research was funded in part through the NIH/NCI Cancer Center Support Grant P30 CA008748.

REFERENCES

1. Genovese G, Kähler AK, Handsaker RE, et al. Clonal hematopoiesis and blood-cancer risk inferred from blood DNA sequence. N Engl J Med 2014;371(26): 2477–87.
2. Jaiswal S, Fontanillas P, Flannick J, et al. Age-related clonal hematopoiesis associated with adverse outcomes. N Engl J Med 2014;371(26):2488–98.
3. Xie M, Lu C, Wang J, et al. Age-related mutations associated with clonal hematopoietic expansion and malignancies. Nat Med 2014;20(12):1472–8.
4. Valent P. ICUS, IDUS, CHIP and CCUS: diagnostic criteria, separation from MDS and clinical implications. Pathobiology 2019;86(1):30–8.
5. Steensma DP, Bejar R, Jaiswal S, et al. Clonal hematopoiesis of indeterminate potential and its distinction from myelodysplastic syndromes. Blood 2015; 126(1):9–16.
6. Khoury JD, Solary E, Abla O, et al. The 5th edition of the World Health Organization classification of haematolymphoid tumours: myeloid and histiocytic/dendritic neoplasms. Leukemia 2022;36(7):1703–19.
7. Hasserjian RP, Orazi A, Orfao A, et al. The international consensus classification of myelodysplastic syndromes and related entities. Virchows Arch 2023;482(1): 39–51.
8. DeZern AE, Malcovati L, Ebert BL. CHIP, CCUS, and other acronyms: definition, implications, and impact on practice. Am Soc Clin Oncol Educ Book 2019;39: 400–10.
9. Valent P, Orazi A, Steensma DP, et al. Proposed minimal diagnostic criteria for myelodysplastic syndromes (MDS) and potential pre-MDS conditions. Oncotarget 2017;8(43):73483–500.
10. Kwok B, Hall JM, Witte JS, et al. MDS-associated somatic mutations and clonal hematopoiesis are common in idiopathic cytopenias of undetermined significance. Blood 2015;126(21):2355–61.
11. Watson CJ, Papula AL, Poon GYP, et al. The evolutionary dynamics and fitness landscape of clonal hematopoiesis. Science 2020;367(6485):1449–54.
12. Acuna-Hidalgo R, Sengul H, Steehouwer M, et al. Ultra-sensitive sequencing identifies high prevalence of clonal hematopoiesis-associated mutations throughout adult life. Am J Hum Genet 2017;101(1):50–64.

13. Young AL, Challen GA, Birmann BM, et al. Clonal haematopoiesis harbouring AML-associated mutations is ubiquitous in healthy adults. Nat Commun 2016;7: 12484.
14. Malcovati L, Gallì A, Travaglino E, et al. Clinical significance of somatic mutation in unexplained blood cytopenia. Blood 2017;129(25):3371–8.
15. Jaiswal S, Natarajan P, Silver AJ, et al. Clonal hematopoiesis and risk of athero- sclerotic cardiovascular disease. N Engl J Med 2017;377(2):111–21.
16. Fuster JJ, MacLauchlan S, Zuriaga MA, et al. Clonal hematopoiesis associated with TET2 deficiency accelerates atherosclerosis development in mice. Science 2017;355(6327):842–7.
17. Tall AR, Fuster JJ. Clonal hematopoiesis in cardiovascular disease and therapeu- tic implications. Nat Cardiovasc Res 2022;1(2):116–24.
18. Zhang Q, Zhao K, Shen Q, et al. Tet2 is required to resolve inflammation by re- cruiting Hdac2 to specifically repress IL-6. Nature 2015;525(7569):389–93.
19. Arber DA, Orazi A, Hasserjian RP, et al. International consensus classification of myeloid neoplasms and acute leukemias: integrating morphologic, clinical, and genomic data. Blood 2022;140(11):1200–28.
20. Parmentier S, Schetelig J, Lorenz K, et al. Assessment of dysplastic hematopoi- esis: lessons from healthy bone marrow donors. Haematologica 2012;97(5): 723–30.
21. Choi E-J, Cho Y-U, Hur E-H, et al. Clinical implications and genetic features of clonal cytopenia of undetermined significance compared to lower-risk myelodys- plastic syndrome. Br J Haematol 2022;198(4):703–12.
22. Gallì A, Todisco G, Catamo E, et al. Relationship between clone metrics and clin- ical outcome in clonal cytopenia. Blood 2021;138(11):965–76.
23. Xie Z, Smith A, Komrokji RS, et al. The Characteristics and prognosis of patients with clonal cytopenias of undetermined significance, including cancer and therapy-related clonal cytopenias. Blood 2022;140(Supplement 1):2887–90.
24. Abelson S, Collord G, Ng SWK, et al. Prediction of acute myeloid leukaemia risk in healthy individuals. Nature 2018;559(7714):400–4.
25. Shanmugam V, Parnes A, Kalyanaraman R, et al. Clinical utility of targeted next- generation sequencing-based screening of peripheral blood in the evaluation of cytopenias. Blood 2019;134(24):2222–5.
26. Baer C, Pohlkamp C, Haferlach C, et al. Molecular patterns in cytopenia patients with or without evidence of myeloid neoplasm-a comparison of 756 cases. Leu- kemia 2018;32(10):2295–8.
27. Ogawa S. Genetics of MDS. Blood 2019;133(10):1049–59.
28. Cargo CA, Rowbotham N, Evans PA, et al. Targeted sequencing identifies pa- tients with preclinical MDS at high risk of disease progression. Blood 2015; 126(21):2362–5.
29. McClure RF, Ewalt MD, Crow J, et al. Clinical significance of DNA variants in chronic myeloid neoplasms: a report of the association for molecular pathology. J Mol Diagn 2018;20(6):717–37.
30. Duncavage EJ, Bagg A, Hasserjian RP, et al. Genomic profiling for clinical deci- sion making in myeloid neoplasms and acute leukemia. Blood 2022;140(21): 2228–47.
31. Kar SP, Quiros PM, Gu M, et al. Genome-wide analyses of 200,453 individuals yield new insights into the causes and consequences of clonal hematopoiesis. Nat Genet 2022;54(8):1155–66.
32. Bolton KL, Ptashkin RN, Gao T, et al. Cancer therapy shapes the fitness land- scape of clonal hematopoiesis. Nat Genet 2020;52(11):1219–26.

33. van Zeventer IA, de Graaf AO, Wouters HJCM, et al. Mutational spectrum and dynamics of clonal hematopoiesis in anemia of older individuals. Blood 2020; 135(14):1161–70.

34. Valent P, Kern W, Hoermann G, et al. Clonal hematopoiesis with oncogenic potential (CHOP): separation from CHIP and roads to AML. Int J Mol Sci 2019;20(3). https://doi.org/10.3390/ijms20030789.

35. Desai P, Mencia-Trinchant N, Savenkov O, et al. Somatic mutations precede acute myeloid leukemia years before diagnosis. Nat Med 2018;24(7):1015–23.

36. Xie Z, Hyun MC, Komrokji RS, et al. Characteristics and clinical outcome of patients with clonal cytopenias of undetermined significance: a large retrospective multi-center international study. Blood 2021;138(Supplement 1):2158.

37. Li M, Binder M, Lasho T, et al. Clinical, molecular, and prognostic comparisons between CCUS and lower-risk MDS: a study of 187 molecularly annotated patients. Blood Adv 2021;5(8):2272–8.

38. Tang G, Medeiros LJ, Wang SA. How I investigate Clonal cytogenetic abnormalities of undetermined significance. Int J Lab Hematol 2018;40(4):385–91.

39. Martin JE, Khalife-Hachem S, Grinda T, et al. Therapy-related myeloid neoplasms following treatment with PARP inhibitors: new molecular insights. Ann Oncol 2021; 32(8):1046–8.

40. Gillis NK, Ball M, Zhang Q, et al. Clonal haemopoiesis and therapy-related myeloid malignancies in elderly patients: a proof-of-concept, case-control study. Lancet Oncol 2017;18(1):112–21.

41. Takahashi K, Wang F, Kantarjian H, et al. Preleukaemic clonal haemopoiesis and risk of therapy-related myeloid neoplasms: a case-control study. Lancet Oncol 2017;18(1):100–11.

42. Wong TN, Ramsingh G, Young AL, et al. Role of TP53 mutations in the origin and evolution of therapy-related acute myeloid leukaemia. Nature 2015;518(7540): 552–5.

43. Shah MV, Mangaonkar AA, Begna KH, et al. Therapy-related clonal cytopenia as a precursor to therapy-related myeloid neoplasms. Blood Cancer J 2022; 12(7):106.

44. Gibson CJ, Lindsley RC, Tchekmedyian V, et al. Clonal hematopoiesis associated with adverse outcomes following autologous stem cell transplantation for non-hodgkin lymphoma. Blood 2016;128(22):986.

45. Lindsley RC, Saber W, Mar BG, et al. Prognostic mutations in myelodysplastic syndrome after stem-cell transplantation. N Engl J Med 2017;376(6):536–47.

46. Coombs CC, Zehir A, Devlin SM, et al. Therapy-related clonal hematopoiesis in patients with non-hematologic cancers is common and associated with adverse clinical outcomes. Cell Stem Cell 2017;21(3):374–82.e4.

47. Takeda J, Miyata T, Kawagoe K, et al. Deficiency of the GPI anchor caused by a somatic mutation of the PIG-A gene in paroxysmal nocturnal hemoglobinuria. Cell 1993;73(4):703–11.

48. Hill A, DeZern AE, Kinoshita T, et al. Paroxysmal nocturnal haemoglobinuria. Nat Rev Dis Primers 2017;3:17028.

49. Kulasekararaj AG, Lazana I. Paroxysmal nocturnal hemoglobinuria: where are we going. Am J Hematol 2023. https://doi.org/10.1002/ajh.26882.

50. Shen W, Clemente MJ, Hosono N, et al. Deep sequencing reveals stepwise mutation acquisition in paroxysmal nocturnal hemoglobinuria. J Clin Invest 2014; 124(10):4529–38.

51. Lee SC-W, Abdel-Wahab O. The mutational landscape of paroxysmal nocturnal hemoglobinuria revealed: new insights into clonal dominance. J Clin Invest 2014;124(10):4227–30.
52. Sun L, Babushok DV. Secondary myelodysplastic syndrome and leukemia in acquired aplastic anemia and paroxysmal nocturnal hemoglobinuria. Blood 2020; 136(1):36–49.
53. Beck DB, Ferrada MA, Sikora KA, et al. Somatic mutations in UBA1 and severe adult-onset autoinflammatory disease. N Engl J Med 2020;383(27):2628–38.
54. Poulter JA, Collins JC, Cargo C, et al. Novel somatic mutations in UBA1 as a cause of VEXAS syndrome. Blood 2021;137(26):3676–81.
55. Georgin-Lavialle S, Terrier B, Guedon AF, et al. Further characterization of clinical and laboratory features in VEXAS syndrome: large-scale analysis of a multicentre case series of 116 French patients. Br J Dermatol 2022;186(3):564–74.
56. Al-Hakim A, Savic S. An update on VEXAS syndrome. Expert Rev Clin Immunol 2023;19(2):203–15.
57. Obiorah IE, Patel BA, Groarke EM, et al. Benign and malignant hematologic manifestations in patients with VEXAS syndrome due to somatic mutations in UBA1. Blood Adv 2021;5(16):3203–15.
58. Templé M, Kosmider O. VEXAS syndrome: a novelty in MDS landscape. Diagnostics 2022;12(7).
59. Kusne Y, Fernandez J, Patnaik MM. Clonal hematopoiesis and VEXAS syndrome: survival of the fittest clones? Semin Hematol 2021;58(4):226–9.
60. Nazha A, Komrokji R, Meggendorfer M, et al. Personalized prediction model to risk stratify patients with myelodysplastic syndromes. J Clin Oncol 2021;39(33): 3737–46.
61. Bersanelli M, Travaglino E, Meggendorfer M, et al. Classification and personalized prognostic assessment on the basis of clinical and genomic features in myelodysplastic syndromes. J Clin Oncol 2021;39(11):1223–33.
62. Bernard E, Tuechler H, Greenberg PL, et al. Molecular international prognostic scoring system for myelodysplastic syndromes. NEJM evid 2022. https://doi.org/10.1056/EVIDoa2200008.
63. Schanz J, Tüchler H, Solé F, et al. New comprehensive cytogenetic scoring system for primary myelodysplastic syndromes (MDS) and oligoblastic acute myeloid leukemia after MDS derived from an international database merge. J Clin Oncol 2012;30(8):820–9.

Morphologic Characteristics of Myelodysplastic Syndromes

Lisa D. Yuen, MD, PhD[a], Robert P. Hasserjian, MD[a],*

KEYWORDS

- Myelodysplastic syndrome • Bone marrow pathology • Ring sideroblasts
- Myeloblast

KEY POINTS

- Morphologic characterization remains a cornerstone in the diagnosis and classification of myelodysplastic syndromes (MDS) in the updated International Consensus Classification (ICC) and 5th edition World Health Organization Classification of Myeloid Neoplasms.
- The presence of dysplasia is one of the key diagnostic criteria required for establishing a diagnosis of MDS, and the percentage of myeloblasts in the blood and bone marrow impacts both disease classification and prognostication.
- Morphologic features also aid in distinguishing MDS from a myriad of other myeloid neoplasms and non-neoplastic mimics. Additional key morphologic features that should be recorded in any MDS case are the bone marrow cellularity and the degree of reticulin fibrosis.
- The morphologic assessment of the bone marrow biopsy, bone marrow aspirate, and peripheral blood smear as it pertains to the diagnosis and up-to-date classification of MDS will be described.
- The implications of the findings on classification and prognosis will also be discussed.

INTRODUCTION

Morphologic characterization remains a cornerstone in the diagnosis and classification of myelodysplastic syndromes (MDS) in the updated International Consensus Classification (ICC) and 5th edition World Health Organization Classification of Myeloid Neoplasms.[1,2] The presence of dysplasia is one of the key diagnostic criteria required for establishing a diagnosis of MDS, and the percentage of myeloblasts in the blood and bone marrow impacts both disease classification and prognostication. Morphologic features also aid in distinguishing MDS from a myriad of other myeloid neoplasms

[a] Department of Pathology-WRN 244, Massachusetts General Hospital, 55 Fruit Street, Boston, MA 02114, USA
* Corresponding author.
E-mail address: rhasserjian@mgh.harvard.edu

Clin Lab Med 43 (2023) 577–596
https://doi.org/10.1016/j.cll.2023.06.003
labmed.theclinics.com
0272-2712/23/© 2023 Elsevier Inc. All rights reserved.

and non-neoplastic mimics. Additional key morphologic features that should be recorded in any MDS case are the bone marrow cellularity and the degree of reticulin fibrosis. In this review, the morphologic assessment of the bone marrow biopsy, bone marrow aspirate, and peripheral blood smear as it pertains to the diagnosis and up-to-date classification of MDS will be described. The implications of the findings on classification and prognosis will also be discussed.

ROLE OF MORPHOLOGY IN DIAGNOSIS

Clinical suspicion for MDS typically arises due to persistent peripheral blood cytopenias. A bone marrow biopsy is often performed when other causes of the abnormal blood counts have been clinically excluded. The presence of dysplastic features affecting at least 10% of the cells in at least one hematopoietic lineage is a main criterion for the diagnosis of MDS. An unexplained increase of blood or bone marrow blasts in a cytopenic patient also supports a diagnosis of MDS, provided other myeloid neoplasms associated with increased blasts (such as acute myeloid leukemia [AML]) are excluded.

COMPONENTS OF THE MORPHOLOGIC EVALUATION

Morphologic evaluation is performed on the bone marrow core biopsy (with or without an accompanying clot section of coagulated bone marrow aspirate), bone marrow aspirate smears, and the peripheral blood smear. The Wright-Giemsa stain is the most important routine stain for cytology that is performed on the bone marrow aspirate and peripheral blood smear. The Perls Prussian-blue stain on the marrow aspirate smear is performed to identify the cytoplasmic iron granules in erythroid precursors; abnormal deposition of iron surrounding the nucleus of erythroid cells defines ring sideroblasts, which occur in a subset of MDS cases and are an indication of erythroid lineage dysplasia. Enzyme cytochemical stains, such as myeloperoxidase or non-specific esterase, can help to highlight granulocytic and monocytic cells respectively, but are no longer routinely used in the workup of MDS. given the wide availability of immunohistochemical stains and flow cytometry. For the core biopsy, routine hematoxylin and eosin (H&E) stain affords the assessment of the marrow cellularity and evaluation of the presence, quantity, and differentiation of each hematopoietic lineage (erythroid, granulocytic, and megakaryocytic); the H&E stain also helps evaluate for extrinsic infiltrates such as lymphoma or carcinoma, which may simulate MDS clinically. Reticulin stain should be performed on all putative MDS cases to grade the degree of fibrosis (on the WHO MF0-3 scale), with a trichrome stain for further evaluation if reticulin is significantly increased (MF grade 2–3). A Giemsa special stain aids in the differentiation of early erythroid precursor cells by staining the cytoplasm of erythroids deeply basophilic, but is not used in all centers. PAS stain can aid in the identification of megakaryocytes, which stain bright pink.

Specimen adequacy and quality of preparation are important factors in both bone marrow biopsies and aspirates, as poorly procured, processed, or stained specimens can preclude morphologic evaluation and impede an accurate diagnosis. In the bone marrow aspirate, an overly thick smear can obscure cell morphology, while poorly prepared smears can lead to numerous traumatized cells with stripped nuclei, rendering the cells unevaluable (**Fig. 1**). Aspicular aspirate smears may consist predominantly or entirely of peripheral blood elements, which precludes accurate evaluation of the marrow composition. The bone marrow aspirate should optimally contain enough cells to perform a 500-nucleated cell differential count, including at least 100 non-erythroid cells.[3] For optimal morphology on the bone marrow biopsy, adequate formalin-based

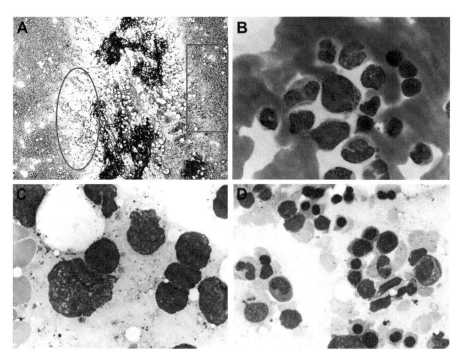

Fig. 1. Artifacts and suboptimal preparations. (*A*) Low power of high-quality BMA showing spicule and well-spread cellular area optimal for counting blasts and evaluating for dysplasia (oval). Thicker areas (box), often farther from the spicule, have obscured cellular morphology. (*B*) Overly thick BMA areas have obscured and poorly preserved cell morphology. (*C*) Overly thin BMA areas have inadequate number of cells and often numerous unevaluable stripped nuclei. (*D*) In the optimal area of aspirate smears, nuclear and cytoplasmic detail is well-displayed in most cells, allowing the optimal enumeration of blasts and dysplasia assessment.

fixation and gentle decalcification are required, as well as thin sectioning of ideally 2um or less. Bone marrow clot sections should contain intact particles of bone marrow, not merely blood clot with scattered hematopoietic cells; an adequate clot section can supplement or even replace a suboptimal core biopsy; in this review, the term "biopsy" applies to both core biopsy and clot section.

The aspirate smear is the gold-standard for evaluating the blast percentage, iron status, and any cytologic dysplasia of myeloid and erythroid cells; megakaryocytic dysplasia is also readily recognized in adequate aspirate smears. The marrow core biopsy is critical to establish the marrow cellularity, the presence and degree of any fibrosis, and architectural organization of hematopoiesis. Cellularity should be adjusted for the patient's age, as normal baseline cellularity decreases progressively with age.[4] Approximately 80% of MDS cases display hypercellularity, while only 10% to 15% are hypocellular for age (see *MDS with hypocellularity or fibrosis*, later in discussion). About 15% of MDS cases show a reticulin grade of 2 or 3 [5]. Architectural disorganization of hematopoiesis in MDS can manifest as abnormally clustered megakaryocytes, lack of well-defined erythroid "islands", or clusters of immature myeloid elements occurring away from bone trabeculae (so-called 'abnormal localization of immature precursors [ALIP], which can be highlighted by CD34 immunostain) (**Fig. 2**). Normally, there are 2 to 4 megakaryocytes per 40x field and they occur singly.

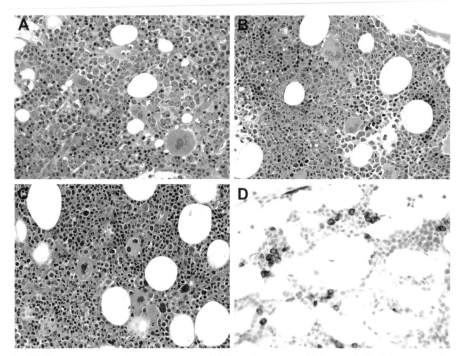

Fig. 2. Bone marrow microarchitecture. (*A*) Reactive erythroid hyperplasia due to autoimmune hemolytic anemia; hypercellularity with enlarged, but maintained erythroid islands and normal megakaryocytes. (*B*) Reactive myeloid hyperplasia due to systemic infection; hypercellularity with immature myeloid elements appropriately located adjacent to bone trabeculum (upper right) and normal megakaryocytes. (*C*) MDS; hypercellularity with the disruption of erythroid islands and abnormal megakaryocytes with simplified nuclei and separated nuclear lobes. (*D*) Abnormal localization of immature precursors (ALIP), representing blasts highlighted by CD34 immunostain.

The ratio of myeloid to erythroid elements in normal marrow is typically 2 to 4:1, with myeloid and erythroid elements forming loose aggregates, and early myeloid elements in reactive hypercellular marrow occurring adjacent to bone trabeculae (**Table 1**).

FEATURES OF DYSPLASIA

Both the ICC and WHO require dysplasia in at least 10% of the cells in at least one hematopoietic lineage to consider a diagnosis of MDS in a cytopenic patient.[1,2,6] **Table 2** lists a summary of dysplastic features in each lineage.

Megakaryocyte dysplasia can be evaluated in both the bone marrow biopsy and aspirate smear. In MDS, the most specific dysplastic features is the "micromegakaryocyte," which is a very small megakaryocyte with a size approximating that of a promyelocyte. Other dysplastic megakaryocytic nuclear features include small size, hypolobated or round/non-lobated nuclei and separated nuclear lobes that are often widely spaced within the cytoplasm (**Fig. 3**A–E). Depending on the sectioning of the tissue, normal megakaryocytes in the core biopsy can display a wide morphologic spectrum, with some cells appearing small and hypo- or mononucleated due to sectioning at the edge of the cell. Unlike micromegakaryocytes, these normal hypolobated megakaryocytes will retain irregular nuclear borders and some connection

Table 1
Important morphologic features which should be included in the pathology report for MDS cases

Specimen	Features	How to Report
BM Biopsy	Cellularity	Percentage, and whether hypocellular for age
BM Biopsy	Megakaryocytes	Distribution and description of cytology
BM Biopsy reticulin stain	Fibrosis	Grade of fibrosis (WHO system, 0–3)
BM Biopsy CD34 stain	Blasts	Estimate of % CD34+ cells of total marrow cells; critical to perform if bone marrow aspirate is suboptimal
BM Aspirate smear	Blasts	% (out of at least 500 nucleated cells)
BM Aspirate smear	Dysplasia	Degree and description of any dysplasia affecting erythroids, granulocytes, or megakaryocytes
BM Aspirate iron stain	Ring sideroblasts	% of nucleated erythroid cells
PB Smear	Counts	Complete blood count and WBC differential
PB Smear	Blasts	% (out of at least 200 nucleated cells)
PB Smear	Granulocytes	Degree and description of any dysplasia

Table 2
Features of dysplasia in hematopoietic cell lineages

	Megakaryocyte	Myeloid	Erythroid
Bone marrow biopsy and aspirate smear	Micromegakaryocytes Hypo-/monolobated nuclei Separated nuclear lobes	Hypogranular cytoplasm Pseudo Pelger-Huet (bilobed nuclei) Abnormal nuclear segmentation Clumping of chromatin Macropolycytes	Nuclear budding Internuclear bridging Cytoplasmic vacuolation Megaloblastoid change Ring sideroblasts
Peripheral blood smea	Platelet anisocytosis Giant platelets Abnormal granulation in platelets	Over 4 nuclear projections	Poikilocytosis Basophilic stippling

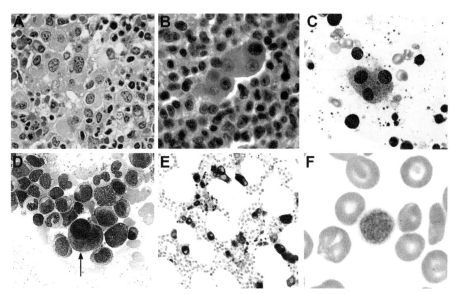

Fig. 3. Dysmegakaryopoiesis. (*A*) Tight clustering of small, hypo- and mononucleated mega-karyocytes. (*B*) Separated nuclear lobes. (*C*) Separated nuclear lobes seen in the bone marrow aspirate smear. (*D*) Micromegakaryocyte (*arrow*), with a nuclear size approximating that of a promyelocyte. (*E*) CD61 immunostain highlights clustered and dysplastic, small megakaryocytes in this case of MDS with multilineage dysplasia. (*F*) Giant platelet in the peripheral blood smear in an MDS case.

between the nuclear lobes (**Fig. 4**). Because of variability in normal megakaryocyte morphology, some studies suggest that 40% (rather than 10%) dysplastic forms is a more appropriate threshold to define dysmegakaryopoiesis; however, 10% bona-fide micromegakaryocytes is considered sufficient to qualify for dysmegakaryopoiesis.[7,8] Megakaryocytes do not typically circulate peripherally, but the observation of platelet anisocytosis, giant platelets, and/or abnormal platelet granulation on the peripheral blood smear can also be indicative of MDS (**Fig. 3**F); however, these platelet abnormalities are not specific for MDS and platelet abnormalities are not counted toward the 10% dysplasia in establishing a diagnosis of MDS.

Dysplasia in the myeloid lineage is most prominent in the maturing granulocytes. A normal granulocyte will have pink granules that are evenly distributed in the cytoplasm and appropriate nuclear segmentation with 3 to 5 lobes. Features of dysgranulopoiesis are best seen on the peripheral blood smear for mature neutrophils and in the bone marrow aspirate for both immature and mature granulocytes. Neutrophils are considered dysplastic if they exhibit hypogranularity of the cytoplasm, which is defined in the 2013 International Working Group on Morphology of Myelodysplastic Syndromes (IWGM-MDS) proposal as at least 2/3 reduction in granules.[9] Pseudo Pelger-Huet cells are granulocytes with symmetrically bilobed nuclei, with the 2 lobes attached by a thin chromatin strand. Other types of neutrophil nuclear dysplasia include abnormal nuclear segmentation (non-lobated round or oval nuclei) and hypersegmentation. Abnormal clumping of chromatin manifests as large blocks of chromatin separated by clear zones. Macropolycytes, or giant neutrophils, can also be seen. The IWGM-MDS proposal suggested that neutrophils with over 4 nuclear projections can also be considered to be dysplastic.[9] **Fig. 5** show examples of features seen in dysgranulopoiesis; any neutrophil with at least one of these morphologic features

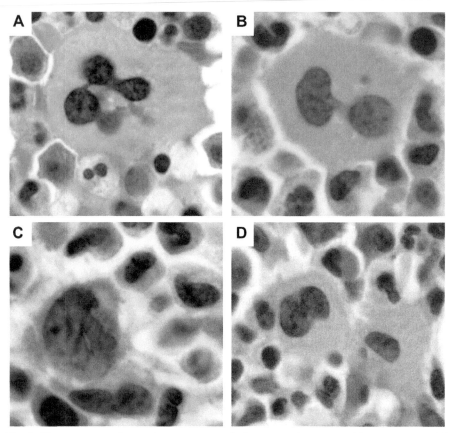

Fig. 4. The spectrum of megakaryocyte morphology seen in a normal bone marrow. (*A*) Typical appearance with large size, lobated nucleus, abundant cytoplasm. (*B*) Smaller size and fewer nuclear lobes visible, however the lobes remain connected. (*C, D*) Small and hypolobated appearance, but nuclear contours are irregular suggesting the appearance is due to sectioning of the cell.

should be considered dysplastic and counted toward the 10% threshold to establish dysplasia within the granulocytic lineage.

Dyserythropoiesis criteria were reviewed and validated by the IWGM-MDS in 2018.[10] Features that are frequently observed in patients with MDS are erythroid nuclear budding, internuclear bridging, multinuclearity, vacuolation, and megaloblastoid change (**Fig. 6**A–E). Nuclear budding is seen as cells with single or multiple buds or lobules projecting off the main erythroid nucleus. Internuclear bridging is defined as a thin strand of chromatin linking two erythroid cells. Vacuolation can present as cytoplasmic vacuoles that are small and round or, more commonly, irregularly shaped and coalescing. Megaloblastoid change is the presence of enlarged erythroblasts with nuclear-cytoplasmic asynchrony such that the maturation stage of the nucleus and cytoplasm are discordant; this is most often manifested as an erythroid cell with cytoplasmic hemoglobinization despite retained immature, relatively dispersed nuclear chromatin. Erythroid abnormalities that are less specific for MDS include cytoplasmic bridging, detached nuclear fragments, and karyorrhexis.[10] Peripheral blood findings in red blood cells include poikilocytosis and basophilic stippling, however, these are

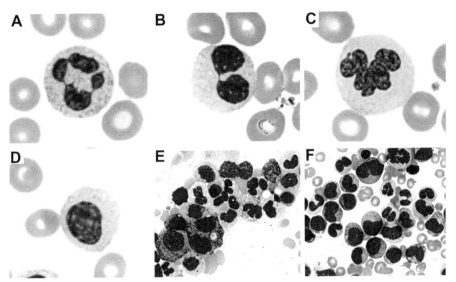

Fig. 5. Dysgranulopoiesis. (*A*) Normal neutrophil with appropriate nuclear segmentation and cytoplasmic granulation. (*B*) Pseudo Pelger-Huet neutrophil with bilobed nucleus and cytoplasmic hypogranulation. (*C*) Hypersegmented dysplastic neutrophil with hypogranular cytoplasm. (*D*) Non-lobated dysplastic neutrophil. (*E, F*) Hypo- and non-lobated myeloid elements with hypogranulation, and uneven granulation in bone marrow aspirate smears from two different patients with MDS.

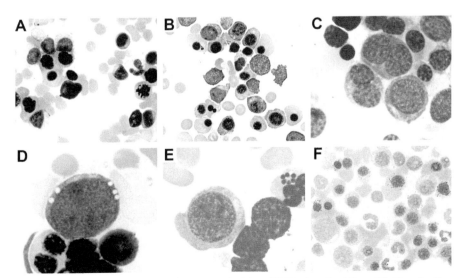

Fig. 6. Dyserythropoiesis. (*A*) Nuclear irregularities. (*B*) Nuclear budding. (*C*) Binucleation. (*D*) Cytoplasmic vacuolation. (*E*) Megaloblastoid changes, manifested by an immature nucleus with fine chromatin surrounded by a hemoglobinized cytoplasm. (*F*) Ring sideroblasts on an iron-stained aspirate smear.

also commonly seen in non-neoplastic conditions. A relatively specific dysplastic finding in erythroid cells is ring sideroblasts (RS), which are defined as erythroblasts with 5 or more siderotic granules surrounding at least one-third of the nuclear circumference[3](**Fig. 6**F). These abnormal granules are formed from abnormal iron accumulation in mitochondria. RS comprising at least 15% of erythroid precursors are strongly supportive of MDS and only rarely occur in non-neoplastic conditions, while rare ring sideroblasts may be seen in reactive conditions such as due to drugs or toxins (see *Classification of MDS*, later in discussion).

DIFFERENTIAL DIAGNOSIS FOR MORPHOLOGIC DYSPLASIA

It is vital to note that dysplastic features in all hematopoietic lineages, but particularly in erythroids, is not specific for MDS and morphologic findings alone are not pathognomonic of neoplastic disease.[11] Morphologic dysplasia can be found in a variety of non-clonal conditions, non-MDS myeloid neoplasms, and even in the bone marrow of healthy donors.[12–14] Thus, unless an unexplained excess of blasts is seen, a diagnosis of MDS should be made with caution or not at all based on the presence of dysplasia alone in cases without clinical information, particularly if results of cytogenetic and molecular genetic testing are not yet available. Potential imitators of MDS include those listed in **Table 3** with examples of dysplastic features illustrated in **Fig. 7**. See chapter 6, later in discussion, for further discussion of mimics of MDS.

When significant dysplasia is seen in the bone marrow of a cytopenic patient, depending on its degree and specificity (for example micromegakaryocytes vs other types of megakaryocytic dysplasia) and the clinical picture (duration of cytopenia and rigorous exclusion of secondary causes of cytopenia), either a presumptive diagnosis of MDS or a descriptive diagnosis may be rendered while awaiting results of ancillary testing. The pathologist must weigh the degree of dysplastic findings in the clinical context: appropriate diagnostic terms that reflect the degree of certainty can include "diagnostic of", "suspicious for", or "raises the possibility of" MDS. Nondefinitive diagnoses can often be confirmed as definitive following receipt of genetic testing indicating a clonal process, and in such cases a clarifying addendum to the report can be issued.

CLASSIFICATION OF MYELODYSPLASTIC SYNDROMES

There have been various classifications of MDS, beginning with the French-American-British (FAB) classification published in 1976 and updated in 1982. The FAB classification was based on clinical and morphologic features as well as the blast percentage.[15] The WHO classification, published in 2001 (3rd edition) and updated in 2008 (4th edition) and 2017 (Revised 4th edition), uses information from clinical findings, morphology, immunophenotype, cytogenetics, and molecular genetics, which has allowed improved risk stratification and targeted therapies for specific entities, such as MDS with isolated del(5q). The recently published International Consensus Classification (ICC)[1] and the proposed 5th edition of the WHO classification[2] have further updated diagnostic criteria, with increased emphasis on genetic classifiers defining MDS subtypes.

IMPACT OF MORPHOLOGIC FINDINGS ON PROGNOSIS AND CLASSIFICATION
Myeloblasts

The assessment of blasts is crucial in the workup of MDS, as increased blasts (5%–19%) in a cytopenic patient is an indication of an aggressive myeloid neoplasm and

Table 3
Non-MDS conditions with morphologic dysplasia

Category	Examples	Morphologic Findings
Nutritional deficiency	Megaloblastic anemia (vit B12/folate deficiency)	Prominent erythroid megaloblastic changes Megaloblastic change in myeloids Hypersegmented neutrophils in PB
Drug/toxin	Chemotherapy, particularly folate antagonists and antimetabolites	Megaloblastic changes
	Recovering marrow after stem cell transplantation	Erythroid and sometimes megakaryocytic dysplasia Circulating blasts, left-shifted myeloids Pseudo-Pelger-Huet cells
	Tacrolimus or Mycopheylate	Ring sideroblasts, erythroid precursor vacuolization
	Alcohol	Dysplasia in all lineages, particularly erythroid
	Heavy metals (arsenic, lead)	Ring sideroblasts
	Antituberculosis drugs (isoniazid)	Ring sideroblasts, erythroid precursor vacuolization
	Zinc toxicity and copper deficiency	Granulocyte precursor vacuolization
Infection	Chronic viral infections (HIV, EBV, HSV, CMV)	Erythroid and megakaryocytic dysplasia
	Parvovirus B19	Dysplasia restricted to erythroid lineage
Autoimmune	Immune thrombocytopenic purpura	Increased number of megakaryocytes with clustering Range of megakaryocyte sizes, including small forms
Other hematologic diseases	Idiopathic dysplasia of undetermined significance	Dysplasia without cytopenia
	MDS/MPN	Dysplasia with leukocytosis or absolute monocytosis
	Primary myelofibrosis	Mimic of fibrotic MDS
	Aplastic anemia	Mimic of hypoplastic MDS
	Paroxysmal nocturnal hemoglobinuria	Erythroid hyperplasia and left shift
	Large granular lymphocytic leukemia	Reactive dysplasia
Constitutional disorders (see Karen M. Chisholm and Sandra D. Bohling's article, "Childhood Myelodysplastic Syndrome," in this issue)	Congenital dyserythropoietic anemias	Erythroid dysplasia
	Congenital sideroblastic anemia	Ring sideroblasts
	Fanconi anemia	Erythroid dysplasia

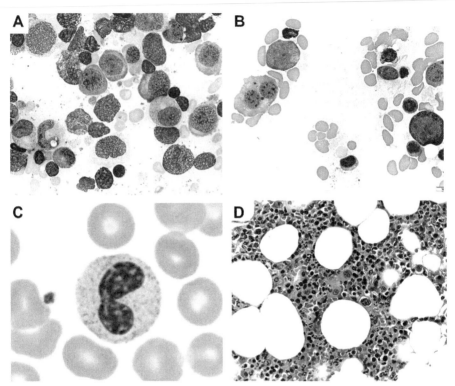

Fig. 7. Morphologic dysplasia in non-MDS conditions. (A) Megaloblastic anemia, with megaloblastoid changes in erythroid and myeloid lineages. (B) Methotrexate toxicity causing left-shifted erythroid maturation and erythroid binucleation. (C) Mycophenylate toxicity, mimicking pseudo-Pelger-Huet change in neutrophil. (D) Immune thrombocytopenic purpura, with increased and small megakaryocytes mimicking those seen in MDS.

places the diagnosis into the MDS with excess blasts (MDS-EB) category. In 2008, the IWGM-MDS group set forth recommendations for the morphologic definition of blast cells and promyelocytes (which are not counted together with blasts) to facilitate accurate blast enumeration.[3] According to their definitions, myeloblasts are cells with a high nuclear to cytoplasmic ratio, easily visible nucleoli, fine nuclear chromatin, variable cytoplasmic basophilia and granulation, and no Golgi zone. The myeloblasts in MDS can be either agranular or granular and may or may not contain Auer rods (**Fig. 8**); of note, any Auer rods identified in blasts in an MDS case mandate classification as MDS-EB2 in the revised 4th edition WHO classification. Promyelocytes have round, oval, or indented and often eccentric nuclei, fine or coarse chromatin, an easily visible nucleolus, and a Golgi zone (**Fig. 8**F). They should be considered dysplastic when cytoplasmic basophilia is reduced, the Golgi zone is absent, and granules are either increased, decreased, and/or irregularly distributed (see **Fig. 8**B). The presence of a discernible Golgi zone (in most cases) and granules helps distinguish dysplastic promyelocytes from true blasts in MDS. Pronormoblasts (large erythroid precursors with round nuclei, finely stippled chromatin, and deeply basophilic cytoplasm, often with perinuclear hof) should not be included in the blast count.

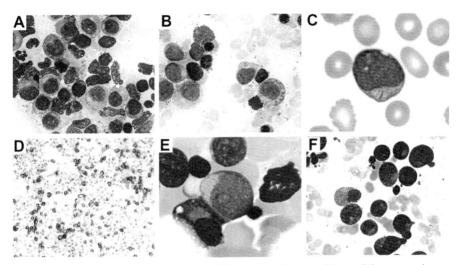

Fig. 8. Myeloblasts and promyelocytes in MDS and reactive conditions. (A) Increased agranular myeloblasts in a case of MDS with excess blasts. (B) Dysplastic promyelocytes with decreased granulation, uneven granulation, and absent Golgi zones in MDS with excess blasts-1, (C) Myeloblast with Auer rod in a case of MDS with excess blasts-2. (D) Immunostain for CD34 shows increased myeloid blasts in a case of MDS with excess blasts-2. (E) Blast in MDS with excess blasts-1, showing fine chromatin, prominent nucleolus, irregular nuclear contour, and scant, agranular cytoplasm. (F) Reactive promyelocytes in a case of myeloid maturation arrest with even granulation and visible Golgi zones.

The blast percentage is a crucial factor in both the classification and prognosis of MDS. The Revised International Prognostic Scoring System (IPSS-R) determined that blast percentage subdivisions at 2%, 5%, and 10%, had an impact on overall survival and leukemia-free survival of patients with MDS.[16] More recently, the IPSS-molecular (IPSS-M) has updated the IPSS-R by the incorporation of molecular genetics alongside the existing IPSS-R variables of blood counts, bone marrow blast percentage, and cytogenetic features. Unlike the IPSS-R, which uses defined blast thresholds, the IPSS-M[17] considers blasts as a continuous variable from 0% to 20%, emphasizing the importance of providing a precise blast percentage (ie, not "blasts are <5%") in the pathology report.

As noted above, a count of at least 500 cells in the bone marrow aspirate smear is important in order to accurately classify and risk stratify MDS cases at the time of initial diagnosis. The bone marrow aspirate differential count is considered the gold standard for blast enumeration, however, aspirates may be poor quality or contaminated by peripheral blood. Even with high-quality and representative marrow aspirates, enumeration of blasts at the lower range (<5% blasts) can lack reproducibility.[18] Furthermore, treated patients with MDS can have variable cellularity and focal areas with clusters of blasts, which conveys a worse prognosis.[5,19,20] Thus the marrow aspirate should be correlated with the core biopsy, including an immunohistochemical (IHC) stain for CD34.[21,22] IHC with CD34 is particularly helpful for enumerating blasts in cases of MDS with fibrosis or hypocellularity, as it can detect a higher blast percentage than the aspirate smear and upstage the patient both in terms of disease category and also the IPSS-R and IPSS-M risk category.[23] Flow cytometric analysis for CD34+ cells is an additional tool for analysis of blasts in MDS, however, it can underestimate the blast count due to lack of universal CD34 expression by blasts and possible hemodilution.[6] Overall, the integration of the aspirate findings, CD34 IHC, and flow cytometric analysis is ideal for the most accurate disease classification and prognosis.

It is also important to review the peripheral smear for any circulating blasts, counting at least 200 nucleated cells. Any blasts seen in the blood of an MDS patient (in the absence of growth factor administration, which may transiently increase blasts in blood and bone marrow) are concerning for progressive disease. Even if the bone marrow blasts are less than 5%, the presence of 2% to 4% blasts in the blood qualifies for a diagnosis of MDS-EB1 and the presence of 5% or more blasts in the blood qualifies for MDS-EB2 in the revised 4th edition WHO classification; the ICC and 5th edition WHO also allow upstaging of patients based on circulating blasts, with the same thresholds as the revised 4th edition WHO. The recognition of circulating blasts is particularly important since these are not taken into account in the IPSS-R and IPSS-M schemes.

Dysplasia

Despite the importance of morphologic dysplasia, assessment can be problematic due to discrepancies in the types of dysplastic features and the threshold required to reach a diagnosis of MDS. As noted previously, even the marrow of healthy volunteers can show dysplasia and marrow specimens can have artifacts leading to difficulty with interpretation. Several studies have proposed dysplasia grading systems in an attempt to improve the accuracy of MDS diagnosis. Liu and colleagues quantified the incidence of specific dysplastic features in MDS cases and discovered that each hematopoietic lineage had a wide range in percentage of dysplastic cells.[24] Della Porta and colleagues also quantified the percentage of hematopoietic cells displaying a specific morphologic abnormality and proposed a morphologic score that incorporated these varying percentages each with a threshold value.[7] As mentioned previously, Matsuda and colleagues proposed that the at least 40% dysmegakaryopoiesis or at least 10% micromegakaryocytes should be present to qualify for dysplasia in the megakaryocyte lineage.[8] Germing and colleagues performed a comprehensive morphologic analysis of over 3000 patients with MDS and also recommended a 40% cutoff for dysmegakaryopoiesis to ensure specificity.[25]

Accurate identification of dysplasia in each lineage has an impact on both diagnostic category and prognosis. The morphologic findings of dysplasia in a single lineage (SLD) versus multiple lineages (MLD) defines distinct diagnostic categories in MDS cases with fewer than 5% blasts,[22] and this distinction has been retained in the ICC as MDS-NOS-SLD and MDS-NOS-MLD disease categories.[1] MDS with single lineage dysplasia (MDS-SLD/MDS-NOS-SLD) are cases with at least 10% dysplasia in only one lineage; of note, the lineages exhibiting dysplasia and cytopenia are not necessarily the same. MDS-SLD carries a relatively favorable prognosis and survival can be similar to age-matched individuals.[26,27] The presence of pancytopenia with dysplasia in only one lineage moved the diagnosis out of MDS-SLD and into MDS, unclassifiable (MDS-U) in the revised 4th edition WHO classification, as these patients have higher risk disease. However, the MDS-U category has been eliminated in both ICC and the WHO 5th edition, and pancytopenia no longer impacts MDS classification in these updated systems.

MDS with multilineage dysplasia (MDS-MLD) must have greater than 10% dysplasia in two or three lineages. The presence of multilineage dysplasia significantly shortens overall survival and leukemia-free survival compared to MDS-SLD. Of note, in the 5th ed. WHO classification, it is considered optional to note single or multilineage dysplasia in cases of MDS with low blasts that lack the defining genetic features of SF3B1 mutation, isolated del(5q), or bi-allelic TP53 inactivation.

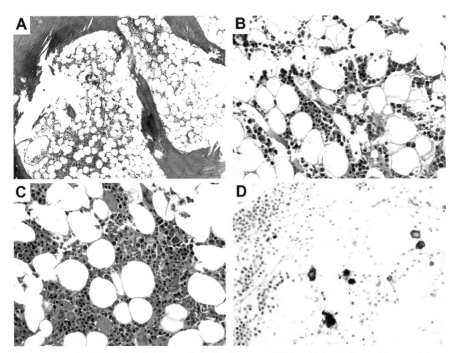

Fig. 9. Hypoplastic MDS. (*A*) Hypocellularity for age (15% cellularity in a 65-year-old patient). (*B, C*) Architectural disruption and megakaryocyte dysplasia. (*D*) CD61 immunostain highlights the dysplastic megakaryocytes.

Ring Sideroblasts

MDS with ring sideroblasts (MDS-RS) is defined in the revised 4th edition WHO as an MDS without excess blasts and having ring sideroblasts identified on an iron stain that comprise at least 15% of the erythroid precursors. Most of these cases are associated with mutated spliceosome gene *SF3B1*, and if such a mutation is identified, this diagnosis can be made with only 5% ring sideroblasts. This category of MDS is important to recognize because patients have a generally favorable prognosis. However, MDS-RS with multilineage dysplasia has worse survival compared to MDS-RS with single-lineage dysplasia, likely due to a higher incidence of mutations in *TP53* and *ASXL1*.[28] More recent data suggest that classifying MDS based on *SF3B1* mutation, rather than ring sideroblasts, better defines a disease category based on biologic features and prognosis; defined as such, single vs multilineage dysplasia have no impact on patient outcome in *SF3B1*-mutated MDS and conversely, ring sideroblasts do not appear to convey prognostic significance in MDS cases lacking *SF3B1* mutation.[29,30] Both ICC and WHO 5th edition now recognize a specific MDS subtype defined by *SF3B1* mutation.

Even in the setting of a newly created SF3B1-mutated MDS entity, performance of an iron stain and enumeration of ring sideroblasts in any putative MDS cases is still essential for the following reasons: 1) Ring sideroblasts represent by definition dysplastic erythroid cells, and count toward the 10% threshold to establish an MDS diagnosis; even smaller numbers of ring sideroblasts can strongly suggest an MDS diagnosis, provided secondary causes of ring sideroblasts are excluded. 2) In cases lacking SF3B1 mutation information, the 5th edition WHO Classification (not the ICC) allows ring sideroblasts comprising $\geq$ 15% of erythroid cells to qualify for a diagnosis of MDS with low blasts and *SF3B1* mutation. 3) Cases with $\geq$ 15% ring sideroblasts but lacking SF3B1 mutation are classified in the morphologically defined entity MDS with low blasts and ring sideroblasts in the 5th edition WHO Classification (not the ICC).

Myelodysplastic Syndromes with Hypocellularity or Fibrosis

In addition to the CD34 IHC assessment, there are several bone marrow core biopsy histologic findings that are important to recognize. In the majority of MDS cases, the marrow specimen is hypercellular for age. However, approximately 10% to 15% of MDS cases are hypocellular for age.[31] Hypocellular (or hypoplastic) MDS is more common in therapy-related disease, in pediatric cases, and in cases arising in patients with prior aplastic anemia. These cases of MDS may be more difficult to diagnose due to fewer cells present for assessment in both the core biopsy and aspirate smears. However, the diagnosis of MDS can be made in hypocellular marrow if there is unambiguous dysplasia or if excess blasts are seen (**Fig. 9**). The prognosis of patients with hypoplastic MDS does not appear to be significantly different from normo/hypercellular MDS[30–34]; however, patients with hypoplastic MDS have some differences in the genetic profile compared to normo/hypercellular MDS and may have a more favorable response to immunosuppression.[35] The 5th edition WHO classification (not the ICC) recognizes hypoplastic MDS as a specific disease category, and thus it is important to specify the bone marrow cellularity and note if the marrow is hypocellular in the

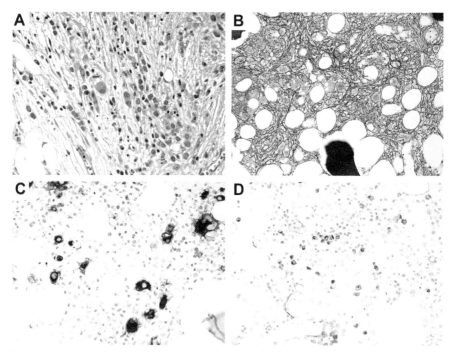

Fig. 10. MDS with increased blasts and fibrosis. (*A*) Abundant background fibrosis with sparse hematopoietic cells, including numerous small, dysplastic megakaryocytes. (*B*) Reticulin stain shows WHO grade 2+ to 3+ fibrosis. (*C*) CD61 immunostain highlights the dysplastic megakaryocytes. (*D*) CD34 immunostain highlights increased blasts, comprising 5% of the cellularity and occurring in clusters.

pathology report. Importantly, a significant subset of hypocellular MDS cases have increased blasts, thus CD34 staining on the bone marrow biopsy is important to perform in this setting; excess blast cases are excluded from the hypoplastic MDS WHO 5th edition entity.

Fibrotic MDS, in which there is an overt bone marrow fibrosis of grade 2 or 3 (in a 3-grade system), comprises 15% of MDS cases. The grading of fibrosis requires the evaluation of a reticulin stain and has been defined as moderate fibrosis with dense and diffusely increased reticulin fibers with extensive intersections and focal thick collagen fibers (grade 2) or severe, dense reticulin fibers mixed with bundles of collagen (identified by trichrome stain) (grade 3).[36] Fibrosis in MDS is associated with poor prognostic factors, including multilineage dysplasia, increased cellularity, and higher transfusion requirements. Patients with MDS with fibrosis have significantly shorter overall and leukemia-free survival compared to patients with MDS with a reticulin grade of 0 or 1 [5]. In fibrotic MDS cases, histologic assessment of a BM core biopsy is critical (**Fig. 10**), as the aspirate smears often are paucicellular and hemodilute. An important differential diagnosis of fibrotic MDS is primary myelofibrosis (PMF); unlike PMF, fibrotic MDS has small and hypolobated megakaryocytes and usually lacks large, hyperchromatic forms. Of note, fibrotic MDS cases may have *JAK2* mutations, and thus this finding does not exclude MDS when evaluating a myeloid neoplasm with bone marrow fibrosis.[37] The 5th edition WHO classification (not the ICC) recognizes MDS fibrosis as a specific disease category of MDS with increased blasts. Thus, reticulin staining (and trichrome staining, if reticulin grade is 2 or 3) should be performed and reported on all MDS cases. Although the WHO 5th edition MDS with fibrosis entity is restricted to cases with excess blasts, it is important to note that grade 2 or 3 bone marrow fibrosis also confers adverse prognosis to low blast MDS subtypes.[37]

SUMMARY

Although the incorporation of information from ancillary testing and molecular findings is increasingly important in newer classification systems, morphologic evaluation of the bone marrow biopsy and aspirate remain the foundation of the diagnosis and classification of MDS. The presence of either morphologic dysplasia or increased blasts is a requirement for establishing a diagnosis of MDS in a cytopenic patient. However, it is important to keep in mind that dysplasia is not a specific finding to MDS and correlation with the patient's clinical presentation must be done. Several factors with significant impact on risk stratification, particularly the blast percentage, but also the number of dysplastic lineages and degree of marrow fibrosis, can only be accurately assessed by morphologic evaluation. Thus, morphologic assessment continues to be critical for the accurate diagnosis, classification, and risk stratification of MDS.

CLINICS CARE POINTS

- Morphologic evaluation of the bone marrow biopsy, aspirate, and peripheral smear remain the foundation of the diagnosis and classification of MDS.
- Dysplasia is not a specific finding for MDS and correlation with the patient's clinical presentation is required.
- Several factors with significant impact on MDS risk stratification (particularly the blast percentage) can only be accurately assessed by morphologic evaluation.

REFERENCES

1. Arber DA, Orazi A, Hasserjian RP. International consensus classification of myeloid neoplasms and acute leukemias: integrating morphologic. Clin Genomic Data 2022;140(11):1200–28.
2. Khoury JD, Solary E. The 5th edition of the World Health organization classification of haematolymphoid tumours: myeloid and histiocytic/dendritic neoplasms. Leukemia 2022;36(7):1703–19.
3. Mufti GJ, Bennett JM, Goasguen J, et al. Diagnosis and classification of myelodysplastic syndrome: international Working Group on Morphology of myelodysplastic syndrome (IWGM-MDS) consensus proposals for the definition and enumeration of myeloblasts and ring sideroblasts. Haematologica 2008;93(11):1712–7.
4. Hartsock RJ, Smith EB, Petty CS. Normal variations with aging of the amount of hematopoietic tissue in bone marrow from the anterior iliac crest. a study made from 177 cases of sudden death examined by necropsy. Am J Clin Pathol 1965;43:326–31.
5. Della Porta MG, Malcovati L, Boveri E, et al. Clinical relevance of bone marrow fibrosis and CD34-positive cell clusters in primary myelodysplastic syndromes. J Clin Oncol 2009;27(5):754–62.
6. Steven H, Swerdlow EC, Lee Harris Nancy, Jaffe Elaine S, et al. WHO classification of Tumours of Haematopoietic and lymphoid tissues (revised. 4th edition. Lyon: IARC Press; 2017.
7. Della Porta MG, Travaglino E, Boveri E, et al. Minimal morphological criteria for defining bone marrow dysplasia: a basis for clinical implementation of WHO classification of myelodysplastic syndromes. Leukemia 2015;29(1):66–75.
8. Matsuda A, Germing U, Jinnai I, et al. Improvement of criteria for refractory cytopenia with multilineage dysplasia according to the WHO classification based on prognostic significance of morphological features in patients with refractory anemia according to the FAB classification. Leukemia 2007;21(4):678–86.
9. Goasguen JE, Bennett JM, Bain BJ, et al. Proposal for refining the definition of dysgranulopoiesis in acute myeloid leukemia and myelodysplastic syndromes. Leuk Res 2014;38(4):447–53.
10. Goasguen JE, Bennett JM, Bain BJ. Dyserythropoiesis in the diagnosis of the myelodysplastic syndromes and other myeloid neoplasms: problem areas. Br J Haematol 2018;182(4):526–33.
11. Steensma DP. Dysplasia has A differential diagnosis: distinguishing genuine myelodysplastic syndromes (MDS) from mimics, imitators, copycats and impostors. Curr Hematol Malig Rep 2012;7(4):310–20.
12. Ramos F, Fernandez-Ferrero S, Suarez D, et al. Myelodysplastic syndrome: a search for minimal diagnostic criteria. Leuk Res 1999;23(3):283–90.
13. Bain BJ. The bone marrow aspirate of healthy subjects. Br J Haematol 1996;94(1):206–9.
14. Parmentier S, Schetelig J, Lorenz K, et al. Assessment of dysplastic hematopoiesis: lessons from healthy bone marrow donors. Haematologica 2012;97(5):723–30.
15. Bennett JM, Catovsky D, Daniel MT, et al. Proposals for the classification of the myelodysplastic syndromes. Br J Haematol 1982;51(2):189–99.
16. Greenberg PL, Tuechler H, Schanz J, et al. Revised international prognostic scoring system for myelodysplastic syndromes. Blood 2012;120(12):2454–65.

17. Bernard E, Tuechler H, Greenberg PL, et al. Molecular international prognostic scoring system for myelodysplastic syndromes. NEJM Evid 2022;1(7). EVIDoa 2200008.
18. Font P, Loscertales J, Soto C, et al. Interobserver variance in myelodysplastic syndromes with less than 5 % bone marrow blasts: unilineage vs. multilineage dysplasia and reproducibility of the threshold of 2 % blasts. Ann Hematol 2015; 94(4):565–73.
19. Horny HP, Sotlar K, Valent P. Diagnostic value of histology and immunohistochemistry in myelodysplastic syndromes. Leuk Res 2007;31(12):1609–16.
20. Valent P, Orazi A, Busche G, et al. Standards and impact of hematopathology in myelodysplastic syndromes (MDS). Oncotarget 2010;1(7):483–96.
21. Malcovati L, Hellstrom-Lindberg E, Bowen D, et al. Diagnosis and treatment of primary myelodysplastic syndromes in adults: recommendations from the European LeukemiaNet. Blood 2013;122(17):2943–64.
22. Arber DA, Orazi A, Hasserjian R, et al. The 2016 revision to the World Health Organization classification of myeloid neoplasms and acute leukemia. Blood 2016; 127(20):2391–405.
23. Saft L, Timar B, Porwit A. Enumeration of CD34+ blasts by immunohistochemistry in bone marrow biopsies from MDS patients may have significant impact on final WHO classification. J Hematopathology 2020;13(2):79–88.
24. Liu D, Chen Z, Xue Y, et al. The significance of bone marrow cell morphology and its correlation with cytogenetic features in the diagnosis of MDS-RA patients. Leuk Res 2009;33(8):1029–38.
25. Germing U, Strupp C, Giagounidis A, et al. Evaluation of dysplasia through detailed cytomorphology in 3156 patients from the Dusseldorf Registry on myelodysplastic syndromes. Leuk Res 2012;36(6):727–34.
26. Maassen A, Strupp C, Giagounidis A, et al. Validation and proposals for a refinement of the WHO 2008 classification of myelodysplastic syndromes without excess of blasts. Leuk Res 2013;37(1):64–70.
27. Verburgh E, Achten R, Louw VJ, et al. A new disease categorization of low-grade myelodysplastic syndromes based on the expression of cytopenia and dysplasia in one versus more than one lineage improves on the WHO classification. Leukemia 2007;21(4):668–77.
28. Malcovati L, Karimi M, Papaemmanuil E, et al. SF3B1 mutation identifies a distinct subset of myelodysplastic syndrome with ring sideroblasts. Blood 2015;126(2):233–41.
29. Malcovati L, Stevenson K, Papaemmanuil E, et al. SF3B1-mutant MDS as a distinct disease subtype: a proposal from the International Working Group for the Prognosis of MDS. Blood 2020;136(2):157–70.
30. Ball S, Singh AM, Ali NA, et al. A product of "clash of titans" or true reflection of disease biology? validation of 2022 who and icc classifications in a large dataset of patients with myelodysplastic syndrome. Blood 2022;140(Supplement 1):1118–20.
31. Tuzuner N, Cox C, Rowe JM, et al. Hypocellular myelodysplastic syndromes (MDS): new proposals. Br J Haematol 1995;91(3):612–7.
32. Yue G, Hao S, Fadare O, et al. Hypocellularity in myelodysplastic syndrome is an independent factor which predicts a favorable outcome. Leuk Res 2008;32(4):553–8.
33. Calabretto G, Attardi E, Teramo A. Hypocellular myelodysplastic syndromes (h-MDS): from clinical description to immunological characterization in the Italian multi-center experience. Leukemai 2022;36(7):1947–50.

34. Bono E, McLornan D, Travaglino E, et al. Clinical, histopathological and molecular characterization of hypoplastic myelodysplastic syndrome. Leukemia 2019; 33(10):2495–505.
35. Nazha A, Seastone D, Radivoyevitch T, et al. Genomic patterns associated with hypoplastic compared to hyperplastic myelodysplastic syndromes. Haematologica 2015;100(11):e434–7.
36. Thiele J, Kvasnicka HM, Facchetti F, et al. European consensus on grading bone marrow fibrosis and assessment of cellularity. Haematologica 2005;90(8):1128–32.
37. Fu B, Jaso JM, Sargent RL, et al. Bone marrow fibrosis in patients with primary myelodysplastic syndromes has prognostic value using current therapies and new risk stratification systems. Mod Pathol 2014;27(5):681–9.

Significance of *SF3B1* Mutations in Myeloid Neoplasms

David C. Gajzer, MD[a], Cecilia C.S. Yeung, MD[a,b],*

KEYWORDS

• *SF3B1* • Mutation • Myeloid • Neoplasm • Tumor • Maematopoiesis

KEY POINTS

- Myelodysplastic syndromes (MDS) form a group of clonal hematopoietic stem cell disorders characterized morphologically by inefficient hematopoiesis, increased apoptosis, dysplasia in one or more of the major myeloid lineages, and peripheral cytopenias.
- The incidence of the MDS is estimated to range from 5.3 to 13.1 cases per population of 100,000.
- Myelodysplastic neoplasm with low blasts and *SF3B1* mutation, previously known as MDS with ring sideroblasts, accounts for 17% of all MDS cases, with an annual incidence of 0.84 cases 100,000 persons, and has a slight male preponderance.
- *SF3B1* mutations are generally more prevalent in low-risk MDS and have been identified as independent predictors of favorable clinical outcome in MDS.

INTRODUCTION

Myelodysplastic syndromes (MDS) form a group of clonal hematopoietic stem cell disorders characterized morphologically by inefficient hematopoiesis, increased apoptosis, dysplasia in one or more of the major myeloid lineages, and peripheral cytopenias. This group of hematopoietic disorders is also characterized by recurrent genetic abnormalities and a multitude of reported clinically significant gene variants (mutations). Although available data vary, the incidence of the myelodysplastic syndromes is estimated to range from 5.3 to 13.1 cases per population of 100,000.[1] Myelodysplastic neoplasm with low blasts and *SF3B1* mutation, previously known as myelodysplastic syndrome with ring sideroblasts, accounts for 17% of all MDS cases,[2,3] with an annual incidence of 0.84 cases per 100,000 persons, and has a slight male preponderance. Of note, 97% of cases with low blasts and at least 15% of cases with ring sideroblasts were reported to carry mutations in splicing genes compared with only 28% of cases with low blasts and no more than 15% of ring sideroblasts.[4]

---

[a] University of Washington, Seattle, WA, USA; [b] Fred Hutch Cancer Center, Seattle, WA, USA
* Corresponding author. 1100 Fairview Avenue North, G7-910, Seattle, WA 98109.
E-mail address: cyeung@fredhutch.org

Clin Lab Med 43 (2023) 597–606
https://doi.org/10.1016/j.cll.2023.07.005
0272-2712/23/© 2023 Elsevier Inc. All rights reserved.

labmed.theclinics.com

SF3B1 mutations are generally more prevalent in low-risk MDS and have been identified as independent predictors of favorable clinical outcome in MDS in most studies.[5,6] *SF3B1* mutations are also present in 20% of patients with myelodysplastic/myeloproliferative neoplasm (MDS/MPN)[7] and in 15% of patients with chronic myeloid leukemia (CML).[8] The clinical consequences of *SF3B1* mutation in MDS are clear, but the functional consequences of these mutations in human cells remain poorly understood. Altered RNA splicing has been suggested as the mechanism underlying the observed phenotypic changes concomitant to splicing factor gene mutations, including *SF3B1*;[9-11] however, the target genes in the hematopoietic stem cell of MDS cases with *SF3B1* mutations are yet to be defined.

SF3B1 GENE

SF3B1 (splicing factor 3b subunit 1) encodes a core component of the RNA splicing mechanism, the U2 small nuclear ribonucleoprotein (**Fig. 1**) involved in the recognition of the branchpoint sequence, and is the most frequently mutated gene in MDS (20–28% of all patients).[12] The spliceosome, a large, dynamic small nuclear ribonucleoprotein composed of small nuclear RNAs associated with proteins, is responsible for removing introns from precursor mRNA (pre-mRNA) and generating mature, spliced mRNAs.[13] A large, diverse, and dynamic protein has been found that interacts with snRNAs to form snRNPs within the spliceosome. SF3B1 contributes a molecular mass of approximately 450 kDa to each snRNP, and it has been demonstrated to play a key role in the recognition and selection of the branch site during splicing by interacting with the pre-mRNA at or near the branch site in a sequence-independent manner, reinforcing stability during the U2 snRNA/BS interaction.[13,14]

The close association between *SF3B1* mutation and the presence of ring sideroblasts is consistent with a causal relationship and makes this the first gene to be strongly associated with a specific morphologic feature of MDS, as reported by Cazzola and colleagues.[7] Ring sideroblasts are erythroid progenitors demonstrating excess mitochondrial iron accumulation morphologically present as at least 5 coarse iron granules encircling one-third or more of the nucleus.[15,16] Regarding hematopoietic progenitors and serologic markers, Ambaglio and colleagues reported significant relationships between the presence of an *SF3B1* mutation and marrow erythroblasts, soluble transferrin receptor, and serum growth differentiation factor 15 overloading.[17] Furthermore, the authors noted that serum hepcidin levels varied considerably, and that the hepcidin-to-ferritin ratio, a measure of adequacy of hepcidin levels relative to body iron stores, correlated inversely with the presence of an *SF3B1* mutation. Based on these findings, it was concluded that patients carrying an *SF3B1* mutation have inappropriately low hepcidin levels, which may explain their propensity to parenchymal iron overloading.

SF3B1 mutations in MDS are primarily heterozygous point mutations. The presence of hotspots (**Fig. 2**) and the absence of nonsense or frameshift mutations in *SF3B1* in patients with MDS suggest that *SF3B1* mutations are likely to be gain/change-of-function mutations. While a heterozygous $Sf3b1^{+/-}$ knockout mouse model has been shown to develop ring sideroblasts, suggesting that haploinsufficiency of *SF3B1* may lead to their formation,[6] recent similar studies have not made this observation.[18,19] Thus, it is yet to be determined whether *SF3B1* mutations found in MDS are loss-of-function mutations or gain/change-of-function mutations.

ALTERNATIVE CLONAL AND NONCLONAL CAUSES OF RING SIDEROBLASTS

It is important to note various causes not involving *SF3B1* mutations can lead to formation of ring sideroblasts. These include congenital and acquired causes. Congenital

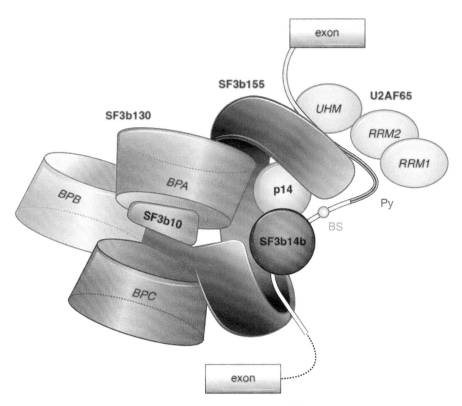

Fig. 1. SF3B1 protein structure and its interaction with collaborative proteins that comprise the core component of the RNA splicing mechanism. U2 small nuclear ribonucleoprotein involved in the recognition of the branchpoint sequence and is the most frequently mutated gene in MDS. (*Adapted from:* Debanjana Maji, Alan Grossfield, Clara L. Kielkopf, Structures of SF3b1 reveal a dynamic Achilles heel of spliceosome assembly: Implications for cancer-associated abnormalities and drug discovery, Biochimica et Biophysica Acta (BBA) - Gene Regulatory Mechanisms, 1862 (11–12), 2019, 194440, https://doi.org/10.1016/j.bbagrm.2019.194440.)

sideroblastic anemia (CSA) is a rare condition that constitutes a diverse class of inherited disorders. Based on the pathophysiology of mitochondrial iron-heme metabolism, CSA-causative genes can be categorized into the following 3 subtypes: heme biosynthesis-associated genes, including 5-aminolevulinate synthase (*ALAS2*), solute carrier family 25 member 38 (*SLC25A38*), and ferrochelatase (*FECH*); Fe–S cluster biosynthesis-associated genes, including ATP binding cassette subfamily B member 7 (*ABCB7*), heat shock protein family A member 9 (*HSPA9*), and glutaredoxin 5 (*GLRX5*), and genes associated with mitochondrial protein synthesis. The most prevalent form of CSA is X-linked sideroblastic anemia (XLSA), which is attributed to mutations in the X-linked erythroid-specific *ALAS2* gene, which encodes the first rate-limiting enzyme in heme biosynthesis.[20,21] *ALAS2* expression is mainly regulated by GATA-binding protein 1 (GATA-1), a master regulator of erythropoiesis.[22]

Among the nonclonal causes of ring sideroblasts, various commonly used drugs are known to be associated with their presence. Although isoniazid and chloramphenicol are most frequently associated with ring sideroblasts, others, such as linezolid, pyrazinamide, penicillamine, cycloserine, fusidic acid, melphalan, busulfan, and triethylenetetramine dihydrochloride, have also been reported. In addition, nutritional

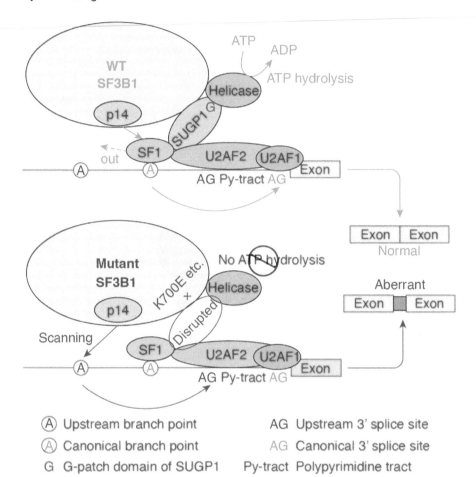

Ⓐ	Upstream branch point	AG	Upstream 3' splice site
Ⓐ	Canonical branch point	AG	Canonical 3' splice site
G	G-patch domain of SUGP1	Py-tract	Polypyrimidine tract

Fig. 2. SF3B1 protein structure showing how hotspot mutation K700E leads to disruption of U2AF2 activity and downstream RNA splicing mechanism. (Jian Zhang, Abdullah M. Ali, Yen K. Lieu, Zhaoqi Liu, Jianchao Gao, Raul Rabadan, Azra Raza, Siddhartha Mukherjee, James L. Manley, Disease-Causing Mutations in SF3B1 Alter Splicing by Disrupting Interaction with SUGP1, Molecular Cell, 76 (1), 2019, 82-95.e7, https://doi.org/10.1016/j.molcel.2019.07.017.)

deficiencies, such as pyridoxine deficiency and copper deficiency, can lead to formation of ring sideroblasts. Moreover, lead intoxication and hypothermia are well-studied environmental causes of ring sideroblasts.[23]

CLASSIFICATION CHANGES FROM 2016 TO NOW

Updates to the World Health Organization (WHO) classification for MDS between the 2016 and 2022 editions primarily placed more emphasis on molecular alterations, and the category of "MDS with ring sideroblasts" was renamed "MDS with *SF3B1* mutation" in 2022. A major change in the WHO fifth edition classification[24] is the adaptation of the term "myelodysplastic neoplasm" (MDN) rather than "myelodysplastic syndrome", although both MDN and MDS are explicitly mentioned as acceptable abbreviations.

Malcovati and colleagues showed in 2 studies that *SF3B1*-mutated MDS represents a distinct subtype of MDS and noted the presence of multilineage dysplasia does not adversely impact prognosis.[25,26] Therefore, the WHO fifth edition further distinction into subcategories of single lineage versus multilineage dysplasia is no longer needed.

In the WHO fifth edition, the main diagnostic criteria for a diagnosis of MDS with *SF3B1* mutation include the presence of dysplasia, low blast count (<5% in BM or <2% in PB), and the presence of an *SF3B1* mutation. In the absence of an *SF3B1* mutation, an exception was retained for the diagnosis of MDS with RS when presence of greater than or equal to 15% ring sideroblasts are seen. Under the WHO fifth edition classification of MDS with *SF3B1* mutation, approximately 17% of MDS cases are expected to fall under this diagnostic category. Further confounding the situation of myeloid disease classification is a second classification system provided by the ICC,[27] where the nomenclature of MDS with *SF3B1* equates to the WHO fifth edition diagnosis of MDS with low blasts and *S3B1* mutation. Cases with *SF3B1* mutations but less than 5% blasts and without significant dysplasia are placed in the new categories of clonal hematopoiesis and clonal cytopenias of undetermined significance (CCUS). Importantly, cases that meet criteria for MDS and carry *SF3B1* mutations or present with ring sideroblasts still need consideration of other diagnostic categories to be ruled out. For instance, cases that show increased blasts above 5% or demonstrate Auer rods should be classified into one of the MDS categories with increased blasts, specifically, those with 5% to 9% as IB-1, and those with 10% to 19% as IB-2. An important distinction in the WHO 5th edition is that the presence of *TP53* mutations or deletion of chromosome 5q supersedes the presence of *SF3B1* mutations in classification considerations, because *TP53* mutations have been shown to portend a poor prognosis. Patients carrying *TP53* mutation(s) in addition to *SF3B1* should undergo further consideration if they qualify for the category of MDS with biallelic (multihit) *TP53* mutation. Detailed discussion of this entity is beyond the scope of this article; however, it is important to mention that patients who are found to carry biallelic *TP53* mutations (two or more *TP53* mutations), as well as those patients with one *TP53* mutation and evidence of *TP53* copy number loss or copy neutral loss of heterozygosity (cnLOH) should be classified as having MDS with biallelic *TP53* inactivation (MDS-biTP53) rather than as MDS with *SF3B1* mutations. Patients demonstrating deletion of the long arm of chromosome 5 (del 5q; MDS with 5q deletion) and carrying a mutation involving the *SF3B1* gene are classified as MDS with chromosome 5q deletion, because the *SF3B1* mutation is considered the probable secondary event.[28] However, conflicting studies have shown that among MDS cases with 5q deletion, patients who also carry an *SF3B1* mutation can expect slightly poorer clinical outcomes.[22,29]

PROGNOSTIC AND TREATMENT IMPLICATIONS OF *SF3B1* MUTATIONS

In 1997, an international MDS risk analysis working group developed the IPSS scoring system accounting for myeloblasts, cytopenia, and cytogenetics.[30] Since the 1997 IPSS, an update was published in 2008[31] and again in 2012, with the IPSS-R, which included an expansion of the cytogenetics groups into 5 subcategories rather than 3.[32] Addition of mutational data into this prognostication system resulted in the IPSS-M system that was published in 2022, in which the molecular mutation profiles of 152 genes were characterized in 2957 patients.[33] Among all MDS subtypes, MDS with low blasts and *SF3B1* mutations have the best outcomes, with most patients demonstrating lower IPSS-R scores[32,34] and, compared with MDS/MPN-RS-T, MDS-SLD-RS cases, have slightly worse clinical outcomes.[34] Given the low risk of leukemic transformation and great outcomes of MDS-LB-SF3B1, treatments have typically been conservative, with management of cytopenias, treating symptoms, improving quality of life, and complication prevention (eg, bleeding, infection, or iron overload).[35] MDS patients with ring sideroblasts who become transfusion dependent are at increased risk of leukemic transformation, and consideration for erythrocyte-stimulating agents or luspatercept[36,37] approved for use in the management of anemia in these contexts is given. Thus, therapy for MDS was limited until the mid-2000s, as the general population had longer life expectancy, and when MDS was recognized as a serious debilitating illness with survival and quality of life implications for a significant proportion of older patients. Azacitidine, a pyrimidine analog causing demethylation, received the first US Food and Drug Administration (FDA) drug approval for use in MDS in 2004.[38] This was followed by FDA approvals of lenalidomide, an immunomodulatory agent,[39] and decitabine, a cytosine analogue and potent inhibitor of DNMT[40] in 2005 and 2006, respectively. In 2020, luspatercept, an inhibitor of SMAD 2/3 signaling,[41] showed in a double-blinded phase 3 clinical trial in very low, low, and intermediate risk MDS with ring sideroblasts lower transfusion requirements when compared with placebo, and obtained FDA approval.[42] It should be noted that despite the current WHO and ICC molecularly driven classification systems, the FDA approval of luspatercept was not based on *SF3B1* status but rather on the presence of ring sideroblasts.[43] In the same year, cedazuridine, which is a cytidine deaminase inhibitor designed to increase levels of decitabine, was approved for use in MDS if given in combination with decitabine.[44]

OTHER MYELOID NEOPLASMS THAT CAN PRESENT WITH RING SIDEROBLASTS OR *SF3B1* MUTATIONS

Although not the focus of this article, the authors will briefly touch on other entities that may present ring with sideroblasts. Ring sideroblasts can have several non-neoplastic etiologies including exposure to toxins and heavy metals (including lead, zinc/copper, and alcohol), drug-related changes, infection, and several genetic syndromes that cause hereditary forms of erythroid dysplasia with ring sideroblasts. Formerly called RARS-T and now classified as MDS/MPN with thrombocytosis and *SF3B1* under the ICC classification and MDN/MPN with *SF3B1* and thrombocytosis under the WHO fifth edition is an entity defined by both myelodysplastic and myeloproliferative features along with demonstration of an *SF3B1* mutation. Despite two different but similar names under the two classification systems, the inclusion criteria for these diagnostic entities are essentially the same: mutations in *SF3B1* (the WHO fifth edition also allows for mutations in other spliceosome genes) or $\geq$ 15% ring sideroblasts, sustained thrombocytosis for 3 months, or the presence of a mutation in *JAK2*, *MPL*, or *CALR* genes.

Another myeloid neoplasm that should be mentioned here is a probable future subcategory of the myelodysplastic/myeloproliferative neoplasm, or overlap syndrome, chronic myelomonocytic leukemia, namely chronic myelomonocytic leukemia with *SF3B1* mutation (termed *SF3B1*[MT] CMML). Wudhikarn and colleagues have defined *SF3B1*[MT] CMML as a CMML subtype with predominant dysplastic features, low frequency of *ASXL1* mutations, higher frequency of JAK2[V61F] mutations, concurrent splicing mutations, and a relatively low risk of progression to acute myeloid leukemia.[45] However, because of its rare occurrence (less than 10% of CMML) and the lack of a clear impact on survival, further validation is needed in a larger cohort of patients before this *SF3B1*[MT] CMML can be recognized as an independent nosologic entity.

SUMMARY

The most significant change in the past 2 years around MDS is the updated prognostic and classification system, which has drawn lines around specific molecular based categories of MDS. When confounding differential diagnoses are ruled out and a diagnosis of MDS with *SF3B1* mutation is confirmed, it carries a favorable prognosis and is amenable to therapies tailored toward patients presenting with ring sideroblasts.

CLINICS CARE POINTS

- Myelodysplastic neoplasm with low blasts and SF3B1 mutation is recognized as a specific WHO diagnostic category, but SF3B1 mutations can be seen in other MDS and MPN neoplasms such as CMML and CML.

- SF3B1 mutations but less than 5% blasts and without significant dysplasia are placed in the new categories of clonal hematopoiesis and clonal cytopenias of undetermined significance (CCUS).

- In the absence of an SF3B1 mutation, an exception to make a diagnosis of MDS with RS was made by the WHO when greater than or equal to 15% ring sideroblasts are seen.

- Cases of MDS with increased blasts above 5% or demonstrate Auer rods should be classified into one of the MDS categories with increased blasts, specifically, those with 5% to 9% as IB-1, and those with 10% to 19% as IB-2.

CONTRIBUTIONS

D.C. Gajzer, drafting manuscript, preparing figures; C.C.S. Yeung, drafting manuscript, preparing figures.

FUNDING

Some of the work for this review article was partially supported by the Fred Hutch Cancer Center Support Grant; P30CA015704.

DISCLOSURE

D.C. Gjzer has disclosures related to the articles. C.C.S. Yeung has received an honorarium for speaking from BMS.

REFERENCES

1. Cogle CR. Incidence and burden of the myelodysplastic syndromes. Curr Hematol Malig Rep 2015;10(3):272–81.
2. Strupp C, Nachtkamp K, Hildebrandt B, et al. New proposals of the WHO working group (2016) for the diagnosis of myelodysplastic syndromes (MDS): characteristics of refined MDS types. Leuk Res 2017;57:78–84.
3. Neukirchen J, Schoonen WM, Strupp C, et al. Incidence and prevalence of myelodysplastic syndromes: data from the Düsseldorf MDS-registry. Leuk Res 2011; 35(12):1591–6.
4. Huber S, Haferlach T, Meggendorfer M, et al. Mutations in spliceosome genes in myelodysplastic neoplasms and their association to ring sideroblasts. Leukemia 2023;37(2):500–2.
5. Malcovati L, Papaemmanuil E, Bowen DT, et al. Chronic myeloid disorders working group of the international cancer genome consortium and of the associazione Italiana per la Ricerca sul cancro Gruppo Italiano Malattie Mieloproliferative. Clinical significance of SF3B1 mutations in myelodysplastic syndromes and myelodysplastic/myeloproliferative neoplasms. Blood 2011;118(24):6239–46.

6. Visconte V, Rogers HJ, Singh J, et al. SF3B1 haploinsufficiency leads to formation of ring sideroblasts in myelodysplastic syndromes. Blood 2012;120(16):3173–86.

7. Cazzola M, Rossi M, Malcovati L. Associazione Italiana per la Ricerca sul Cancro Gruppo Italiano Malattie Mieloproliferative. Biologic and clinical significance of somatic mutations of SF3B1 in myeloid and lymphoid neoplasms. Blood 2013; 121(2):260–9.

8. Tang AD, Soulette CM, van Baren MJ, et al. Full-length transcript characterization of SF3B1 mutation in chronic lymphocytic leukemia reveals downregulation of retained introns. Nat Commun 2020;11(1):1438.

9. Yoshida K, Sanada M, Shiraishi Y, et al. Frequent pathway mutations of splicing machinery in myelodysplasia. Nature 2011;478(7367):64–9.

10. Damm F, Thol F, Kosmider O, et al. SF3B1 mutations in myelodysplastic syndromes: clinical associations and prognostic implications. Leukemia 2012; 26(5):1137–40.

11. Visconte V, Makishima H, Jankowska A, et al. SF3B1, a splicing factor is frequently mutated in refractory anemia with ring sideroblasts. Leukemia 2012; 26(3):542–5.

12. Papaemmanuil E, Gerstung M, Malcovati L, et al. Chronic Myeloid Disorders Working Group of the International Cancer Genome Consortium. Clinical and biological implications of driver mutations in myelodysplastic syndromes. Blood 2013;122(22):3616–27, quiz 3699.

13. Zhou Z, Gong Q, Wang Y, et al. The biological function and clinical significance of SF3B1 mutations in cancer. Biomark Res 2020;8:38.

14. Krämer A. The structure and function of proteins involved in mammalian pre-mRNA splicing. Annu Rev Biochem 1996;65:367–409.

15. Mufti GJ, Bennett JM, Goasguen J, et al. International Working Group on Morphology of Myelodysplastic Syndrome. Diagnosis and classification of myelodysplastic syndrome: International Working Group on Morphology of Myelodysplastic Syndrome (IWGM-MDS) consensus proposals for the definition and enumeration of myeloblasts and ring sideroblasts. Haematologica 2008;93(11): 1712–7.

16. Dolatshad H, Pellagatti A, Fernandez-Mercado M, et al. Disruption of SF3B1 results in deregulated expression and splicing of key genes and pathways in myelodysplastic syndrome hematopoietic stem and progenitor cells. Leukemia 2015; 29(5):1092–103. Erratum in: Leukemia. 2015 Aug;29(8):1798. PMID: 25428262; PMCID: PMC4430703.

17. Ambaglio I, Malcovati L, Papaemmanuil E, et al. Inappropriately low hepcidin levels in patients with myelodysplastic syndrome carrying a somatic mutation of SF3B1. Haematologica 2013;98(3):420–3.

18. Matsunawa M, Yamamoto R, Sanada M, et al. Haploinsufficiency of Sf3b1 leads to compromised stem cell function but not to myelodysplasia. Leukemia 2014; 28(9):1844–50.

19. Wang C, Sashida G, Saraya A, et al. Depletion of Sf3b1 impairs proliferative capacity of hematopoietic stem cells but is not sufficient to induce myelodysplasia. Blood 2014;123(21):3336–43.

20. Fujiwara T, Harigae H. Molecular pathophysiology and genetic mutations in congenital sideroblastic anemia. Free Radic Biol Med 2019;133:179–85.

21. Harigae H, Furuyama K. Hereditary sideroblastic anemia: pathophysiology and gene mutations. Int J Hematol 2010;92(3):425–31.

22. Fujiwara T, O'Geen H, Keles S, et al. Discovering hematopoietic mechanisms through genome-wide analysis of GATA factor chromatin occupancy. Mol Cell 2009;36(4):667–81.

23. Rodriguez-Sevilla JJ, Calvo X, Arenillas L. Causes and pathophysiology of acquired sideroblastic anemia. Genes 2022;13(9):1562.

24. Citation: WHO Classification of Tumours Editorial Board. Haematolymphoid tumours (Internet; beta version ahead of print). Lyon (France): International Agency for Research on Cancer; 2022 (cited YYYY Mmm D). (WHO classification of tumours series, 5th ed.; vol. 11). Available at: https://tumourclassification.iarc. who.int/chapters/63.

25. Malcovati L, Stevenson K, Papaemmanuil E, et al. SF3B1-mutant MDS as a distinct disease subtype: a proposal from the International Working Group for the Prognosis of MDS. Blood 2020;136(2):157–70. Erratum in: Blood 2021;137(21):3003. PMID: 32347921; PMCID: PMC7362582.

26. Malcovati L, Karimi M, Papaemmanuil E, et al. SF3B1 mutation identifies a distinct subset of myelodysplastic syndrome with ring sideroblasts. Blood 2015;126(2): 233–41.

27. Arber DA, Orazi A, Hasserjian RP, et al. International consensus classification of myeloid neoplasms and acute leukemias: integrating morphologic, clinical, and genomic data. Blood 2022;140(11):1200–28.

28. Woll PS, Kjällquist U, Chowdhury O, et al. Myelodysplastic syndromes are propagated by rare and distinct human cancer stem cells in vivo. Cancer Cell 2014 Jun 16;25(6):794–808. Erratum in: Cancer Cell 2014;25(6):861. Erratum in: Cancer Cell 2015;27(4):603-5. PMID: 24835589.

29. Meggendorfer M, Haferlach C, Kern W, et al. Molecular analysis of myelodysplastic syndrome with isolated deletion of the long arm of chromosome 5 reveals a specific spectrum of molecular mutations with prognostic impact: a study on 123 patients and 27 genes. Haematologica 2017;102(9):1502–10.

30. Greenberg P, Cox C, LeBeau MM, et al. International scoring system for evaluating prognosis in myelodysplastic syndromes. Blood 1997;89(6):2079–88. Erratum in: Blood 1998;91(3):1100. PMID: 9058730.

31. Kao JM, McMillan A, Greenberg PL. International MDS risk analysis workshop (IMRAW)/IPSS reanalyzed: impact of cytopenias on clinical outcomes in myelodysplastic syndromes. Am J Hematol 2008;83(10):765–70.

32. Greenberg PL, Tuechler H, Schanz J, et al. Revised international prognostic scoring system for myelodysplastic syndromes. Blood 2012;120(12):2454–65.

33. Bernard E, Tuechler H, Greenberg PL, et al. Molecular international prognostic scoring system for myelodysplastic syndromes. NEJM Evid 2022;1(7).

34. Patnaik MM, Tefferi A. Myelodysplastic syndromes with ring sideroblasts (MDS-RS) and MDS/myeloproliferative neoplasm with RS and thrombocytosis (MDS/MPN-RS-T) - "2021 update on diagnosis, risk-stratification, and management.". Am J Hematol 2021;96(3):379–94.

35. Platzbecker U. Treatment of MDS. Blood 2019;133(10):1096–107.

36. Platzbecker U, Germing U, Götze KS, et al. Luspatercept for the treatment of anaemia in patients with lower-risk myelodysplastic syndromes (PACE-MDS): a multicentre, open-label phase 2 dose-finding study with long-term extension study. Lancet Oncol 2017;18(10):1338–47. Erratum in: Lancet Oncol. 2017;18(10):e562. PMID: 28870615.

37. Fenaux P, Platzbecker U, Mufti GJ, et al. Luspatercept in patients with lower-risk myelodysplastic syndromes. N Engl J Med 2020;382(2):140–51.

38. Siddiqui MA, Scott LJ. Azacitidine: in myelodysplastic syndromes. Drugs 2005; 65(13):1781–9 ; discussion 1790-1.

39. Kotla V, Goel S, Nischal S, et al. Mechanism of action of lenalidomide in hematological malignancies. J Hematol Oncol 2009;2:36.

40. Plimack ER, Kantarjian HM, Issa JP. Decitabine and its role in the treatment of hematopoietic malignancies. Leuk Lymphoma 2007;48(8):1472–81.

41. Suragani RN, Cadena SM, Cawley SM, et al. Transforming growth factor-β superfamily ligand trap ACE-536 corrects anemia by promoting late-stage erythropoiesis. Nat Med 2014;20(4):408–14.

42. Fenaux P, Platzbecker U, Mufti GJ, et al. Luspatercept in Patients with Lower-Risk Myelodysplastic Syndromes. N Engl J Med 2020;382(2):140–51.

43. From: Luspatercept-aamt approved for anemia in adults with MDS, based on FDA press release from April 3rd, 2020. Available at: https://www.ashclinicalnews.org/news/latest-and-greatest/luspatercept-aamt-approved-anemia-adults-mds/.

44. Garcia-Manero G, Griffiths EA, Steensma DP, et al. Oral cedazuridine/decitabine for MDS and CMML: a phase 2 pharmacokinetic/pharmacodynamic randomized crossover study. Blood 2020;136(6):674–83.

45. Wudhikarn K, Loghavi S, Mangaonkar AA, et al. SF3B1-mutant CMML defines a predominantly dysplastic CMML subtype with a superior acute leukemia-free survival. Blood Adv 2020;4(22):5716–21.

Diagnosis and Classification of Myelodysplastic Syndromes with Mutated *TP53*

Alexa J. Siddon, MD[a,b],*, Olga K. Weinberg, MD[c]

KEYWORDS

- *TP53* • Mutations • Myelodysplastic syndromes • Myelodysplasia
- Next generation sequencing • Cytogenetics • Prognosis

KEY POINTS

- MDS is becoming increasingly genetically defined with both the WHO-HAEM5 and ICC recognizing *TP53*-defining mutations in the classification of MDS.
- The incorporation of high-throughput sequencing technologies such as NGS into routine workflows has helped to make the molecular characterization of MDS standard of care.
- Genomic findings are playing a significant role in myeloid disease prognostication including risk stratification and predicting overall survival with the new IPSS-M scoring system as compared to the prior IPSS-R.

INTRODUCTION

Myelodysplastic syndromes/neoplasms (MDS), are a group of clonal hematopoietic stem cell disorders characterized by ineffective hematopoiesis leading to peripheral cytopenias, dysplastic changes in one or more cellular lineages, and an increased risk of progression to acute myeloid leukemia (AML).[1,2] Due to the heterogeneity of clinical features, risk of disease progression, and optimal therapeutic regimens, correctly diagnosing the subtype of MDS is critical.[3] In recent years there been a tremendous influx of genetic information that has led to MDS becoming increasingly genetically defined.[4] Recently, there have been two parallel revisions to the classification of MDS: the International Consensus Classification (ICC), written by a Clinical Advisory Committee convened by the Society for Hematopathology and the European Association for Haematopathology, and the 5th edition of the World Health

[a] Department of Laboratory Medicine, Yale School of Medicine, 330 Cedar Street, PO Box 208035, New Haven, CT 06520, USA; [b] Department of Pathology, Yale School of Medicine, 330 Cedar Street, PO Box 208035, New Haven, CT 06520, USA; [c] Department of Pathology, University of Texas Southwestern Medical Center, BioCenter, 2230 Inwood Road, EB03.220G, Dallas, TX 75235, USA
* Corresponding author. 330 Cedar Street, PO Box 208035, New Haven, CT 06520.
E-mail address: alexa.siddon@yale.edu

Clin Lab Med 43 (2023) 607–614
https://doi.org/10.1016/j.cll.2023.07.004
0272-2712/23/© 2023 Elsevier Inc. All rights reserved.

Organization Classification of Haematolymphoid Tumours (WHO-HAEM5).[1,2] These updates highlight the increasing understanding of the genetic underpinings of MDS, which was previously classified by largely by morphologic characteristics or risk of progression to AML. We now appreciate that the evolution to AML may represent a spectrum of disease and genetic abnormalities may be as important (if not more important) than blast count.

TP53, also known as the guardian of the genome, is a tumor suppressor gene that is essential for DNA damage response and repair, in addition to facilitating genome stability.[5] Further, it is the most commonly mutated gene in human malignancies.[6] TP53 mutations are frequent in MDS and portend a particularly adverse prognosis. This review will focus on TP53 mutations in the context of MDS, including their prevalence, with a focus on the diagnostic aspects of TP53-mutated disease.

BIOLOGY OF TP53 IN HEMATOPOIESIS

The tumor suppressor gene TP53 is located on chromosome 17p13.1, with 11 of its 13 exons involved in coding the p53 protein. The TP53 protein product plays critical roles in the induction of apoptosis, maintenance of cell-cycle regulation, and genome stability to prevent oncogenesis.[5,6] The protein activity is tightly regulated on multiple levels, including transcriptional, post-transcriptional, and post-translational mechanisms, to ensure its proper function in response to cellular stress and DNA damage.[7] The loss of functional p53 can promote malignant transformation, as cells with DNA damage or other oncogenic mutations may continue to divide and evade programmed cell death.[5–8]

The role of TP53 in normal hematopoiesis is multifaceted. It participates in the maintenance of hematopoietic stem cells by regulating their self-renewal and differentiation capacities. The protein p53 acts as a sensor of cellular stress, including DNA damage, hypoxia, and oncogene activation. Upon the detection of such stress signals, p53 activates transcriptional programs that induce cell cycle arrest, DNA repair, or apoptosis, depending on the severity of the damage.[5,6] In normal hematopoiesis this ensures the elimination of damaged or aberrant cells, preventing the propagation of genetic abnormalities and the development of myeloid malignancies.[9]

Several studies have highlighted the importance of TP53 in the regulation of hematopoietic stem cell function. Loss or mutation of TP53 has been associated with the development of MDS and AML. The genomic instability caused by TP53 alterations can result increased hematopoietic stem cell self-renewal and resistance to apoptosis, which may in turn promote the expansion of preleukemic or leukemic clones.[9,10] Therefore, the proper functioning of TP53 is crucial for maintaining the delicate balance between self-renewal and differentiation in normal hematopoiesis, preventing the emergence of myeloid disorders.[11]

TP53 MUTATIONS IN MYELODYSPLASTIC SYNDROMES AND ACUTE MYELOID LEUKEMIA

While TP53 mutations are seen in up to 50% of solid tumor malignancies, it is estimated that TP53 is mutated in only about 5-10% of primary MDS and AML cases.[6,12–14] As MDS and AML are increasingly understood to represent a spectrum of disease, they are often referred to together as one entity. Further, they are frequently associated with complex karyotypes and secondary myeloid neoplasms, with only 1% of normal karyotype MDS and AML cases having TP53 mutations, 40-50% of therapy-related or secondary myeloid neoplasms, and up to 83% of complex karyotype patients having TP53 mutations.[15–17] It is noted that there is a significantly increased incidence of *TP53*-mutated MDS and AML in elderly patients and those exposed to cytotoxic chemotherapy or environmental toxins,[18] however the mechanisms that cause *TP53* mutation enrichment in following cytotoxic therapy are not well understood. It is hypothesized that prior cytotoxic therapy or radiation does not induce *TP53* mutations, but rather preexisting progenitor cells harboring mutations are resistant to DNA damage and clonally expand. Understanding the clinical and molecular characteristics of *TP53*-mutated MDS and AML is of critical importance as its poor prognosis and resistance to conventional chemotherapy is well documented.[19]

Similar to solid tumors, the *TP53* mutations found in MDS and AML are located in exons 4 to 8 of the gene and encode the DNA binding domain.[20] While up to 70-75% of *TP53* mutations in MDS and AML are missense mutations centered around several hotspots but ultimately spanning the gene, there are also structural abnormalities leading various levels of protein functionality.[21] *TP53* missense mutations at the hotspots of codons R175, R248, and R273 typically result in loss of transcriptional activity, leading to the downregulation of apoptosis and upregulation of genes associated with cell cycle arrest when presented with DNA damage.[13] In "non-hotspot" mutations there may be some retention of function, or only partial loss-of-function, and p53 may have some transcriptional activity.[22] The missense mutations of *TP53* in MDS lead to a dominant negative effect, in which the mutations adversely affects the wild-type copy of the gene, and the cell functionally losses both genes.[23] An additional type of *TP53* aberrancy is Loss of Heterozygosity (LOH), in which the wild-type copy of a *TP53* allele is lost and replaced with a second copy of the mutated allelic. In the case of LOH the cell is then homozygous for the mutated *TP53*. For functional purposes, this is the equivalent to a structural deletion of chromosome 17 or 17p.[24] This concept is important for the classification and laboratory identification of *TP53*-mutated MDS.

Current Classification of TP53-Mutated Myelodysplastic Syndromes

Until 2022, the classification of MDS did not have a specific category designated for *TP53*-defined disease. In the World Health Organization (WHO) revised 4th edition MDS was largely designated by morphology and blast count, with the only exception being MDS with isolated del(5q).[25]

In 2022, two parallel classification schemes were published: the ICC and the WHO-HAEM5, the latter of which renamed MDS to myelodysplastic neoplasms (but retained the acronym MDS).[1,2] Both the ICC and WHO-HAEM5 updated their guidelines to include the distinct classification of *TP53*-mutated MDS which supercedes all other types of MDS. One important highlight of these updates is the ICC separates *TP53*-mutated disease into three specific entities encompassing the umbrella category of "myeloid neoplasms with mutated *TP53*": MDS, MDS/AML, and AML, based primarily on bone marrow blast percentages of 0-9%, 10-20%, and >20% respectively. The WHO-HAEM5 designates *TP53*-mutated MDS as having the traditional 0-19% blasts. In addition, for both the ICC and WHO-HAEM5 *TP53*-mutated MDS now requires the presence of multiple *TP53* "hits" – defined as a mutation in at least one *TP53* allele with a variant allele frequency (VAF) ≥10% by next-generation sequencing (NGS) in combination with either (A) a second *TP53* mutation or (B) loss of a 17p13.1 locus as detected by traditional karyotype, fluorescence in situ hybridization (FISH), or LOH. As LOH is not routinely performed at many laboratories (see next section), the WHO-HAEM5 and ICC infer a multiple hit *TP53* status with a >50% VAF by NGS.[1,2] Further, the ICC also allows the equivalent diagnosis of multiple *TP53* hits if there is one mutation and a complex karyotype (defined as ≥3 abnormalities), even in the absence of loss of 17p, as there is such a strong correlation between complex karyotype and multiple *TP53* hits.[1,17,26] The ICC uses the terminology "multi-hit" while WHO-HAEM5 refers to "biallelic inactivation." In the ICC classifications with >10% blasts (MDS/AML with mutated *TP53* and AML with mutated *TP53*) only one somatic *TP53* mutation is needed as the prognosis is similar to multihit *TP53* status (**Fig. 1**). This classification was proposed to highlight that *TP53*-mutated disease has similar dismal prognostic outcomes regardless of AML or MDS diagnosis or blast percentage, and as such, necessitates similar therapeutic considerations. In addition to *de novo* or secondary MDS and AML the WHO-HAEM5 and ICC both recognize germline *TP53* mutations associated with Li-Fraumeni syndrome.[1,2]

Laboratory Analysis of TP53

In order to assess for the multihit status of *TP53*-mutated MDS, as described by the WHO-HAEM5 and ICC, blood or marrow is typically interrogated by multiple different molecular and genetic modalities. The importance of NGS takes a front and center role in *TP53*-mutated MDS, as at least one allele needs to have a mutation with a VAF $\geq$10%.[1,2]

NGS technologies have become more accessible as well as more routinely performed within clinical laboratories. Targeted gene panels have allowed for the evaluation of many genes with relatively high sensitivity, assessing millions of sequencing reaction in parallel. Further, as up to 80% of all MDS cases contain somatic mutations,[4] assessing numerous genes simultaneously is of utmost importance. Most commonly, NGS is designed to detect missense variants as well as small insertions and deletions.[27] Although less commonly, some NGS panels can be designed to identify gene fusions/translocations, copy number variation, and even gene expression and methylation. As a semi-quantitative methodology, NGS shows the number of mutated reads at any position divided by the total reads in that position as a VAF, with analytical sensitivity typically around 2-5%.[27] The information from NGS panels has been tremendous in the understanding, diagnosis, and classification of disease in patients with MDS and AML. Further, it has allowed for molecular monitoring, leading to refined prognostication and therapeutic decision-making.

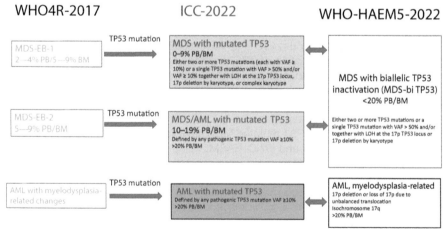

Fig. 1. Comparison of the classifications of TP53-mutated myeloid neoplasms in the classifications including WHO4R-2017, ICC, and WHO-HAEM5. AML, acute myeloid leukemia; BM, bone marrow; LOH, loss of heterozygosity; MDS, myelodysplastic syndrome/neoplasm; PB, peripheral blood.

While Sanger sequencing can detect variants within a single gene such as *TP53*, and is relatively inexpensive, it may not detect smaller clones as the mutation must be present in >20% of cells.[28] Further, it can take as long to perform as an NGS panel and in patients newly being evaluated for MDS, larger panels assessing multiple genes is likely to be more useful.

Cytogenetic analysis continues to be an essential component in the diagnostic evaluation of myeloid malignancies, including *TP53*-mutated MDS. Conventional cytogenetics (ie, karyotyping by chromosomal banding) remains the gold standard technique for chromosomal abnormalities. However, karyotyping requires successful cell division from the neoplastic clone (with ≥20 metaphases) and has a relatively low sensitivity. Aberrations of chromosome 17 are detected in 2–5% of patients with MDS or *de novo* AML, and in over 30% of therapy-related myeloid neoplasms using metaphase G-banding.[18,29] In addition to chromosome 17 alterations, metaphase analysis is important for the detection of additional genetic abnormalities, such as the complex karyotype that is frequently found in conjunction with *TP53* mutations. The limitations of conventional karyotyping include having to culture live cells in vitro, the low analytical sensitivity of having abnormalities present in at least 5-10% of cells that grew, and a turnaround time of up to 3 weeks.[27]

Fluorescence in situ hybridization (FISH) is a faster and more sensitive method to detect chromosome abnormalities and it is performed on interphase cells that do not require cell division.[27] However, probes must be chosen to assess targeted gene regions, rather than assessing the full array of chromosomes that is accomplished by karyotype. FISH is recommended by both the National Comprehensive Cancer Network (NCCN) in the event that conventional cytogenetics cannot be obtained or the cells do not grow.[30]

Finally, chromosomal microarrays (CMAs) are another methodology that can be used to assess copy number-neutral LOH. LOH typically requires a higher chromosomal resolution than conventional karyotyping and do not require the targeted probes of FISH. CMAs have a longer turnaround time than either FISH or karyotyping, and may not be routinely performed.[27]

While there are additional molecular and genetic testing modalities to assess *TP53* mutations, they are currently not standard of care and/or not widely available. These include comparative genomic hybridization, optical genome mapping, single nucleotide polymorphism arrays, and whole exome/transcriptome sequencing.

Prognostic Considerations

Multi-hit *TP53* mutations in MDS are associated with poor clinical outcomes, including higher risk of disease progression to overt AML, resistance to chemotherapy, and a higher risk of relapse and shorter progression-free survival an overall survival following transplant.[13] Additionally, the ICC de-emphasizes the blast count by incorporating the MDS/AML category requiring only one *TP53* mutation, similar to that of overt *TP53*-mutated AML.[1] For more than ten years, the main tool for risk stratification in MDS has been the Revised Prognostic Scoring System (IPSS-R). The IPSS-R uses the following clinical factors to assign a prognostic risk category to patients with MDS: hemoglobin level, absolute neutrophil count, platelet count, and blast percentage in addition to select cytogenetic abnormalities.[31] It was observed that the IPSS-R had a limitation as a subset of patients assigned low risk experienced inferior outcomes when compared to other low risk patients.[32] With the increasing knowledge about the mutational landscape of MDS, it was shown that adding mutational data to the IPSS-R could provide superior prognostication.[4,33] In 2022, the International Working Group for Prognosis in MDS published the International Prognostic Scoring System-

Molecular (IPSS-M), which added a molecular profile of numerous genes mutated in MDS to the IPSS-R, to include multi-hit status of *TP53*. Scoring produces a number on a continuous index which provides prognostic information for estimated leukemia-free survival, risk of leukemic transformation, and overall survival.[34] Kewan and colleagues[35] then validated the IPSS-M using a sample of 1281 patients with MDS, which demonstrated the ability of the IPSS-M to further risk stratify patients based on genetic features, who were previously assigned to the low risk IPSS-R prognostic group based on clinical and cytogenetic factors alone. Further validation in diverse clinical scenarios is required to establish the general clinical utility of this tool.

As prognostication becomes better refined, and new potential molecular targets are identified opportunities for personalized, targeted therapy for this disease will emerge. While there are no current approved drugs for *TP53*-mutated MDS, the combination of molecularly defined category and the blurring of strict classification based on blast count may direct patients toward clinical trials, as *TP53*-mutated MDS has a dismal clinical outcome.

SUMMARY

In conclusion, *TP53* mutations are a relatively common and poor prognostic feature in MDS. The mechanisms underlying the adverse clinical effects of *TP53* mutations in MDS are multifactorial, including increased genomic instability, abnormal cell proliferation, and resistance to apoptosis. The prevalence of *TP53* mutations varies depending on the MDS subtype, with higher rates seen in secondary MDS and cases with complex karyotype.[16,17] *TP53* mutations are associated with decreased overall survival, making them a critical factor to identify when managing patients with MDS. The incredible importance of genetic mutations in the pathogenesis, classification, and prognosis of MDS have become more apparent in recent years following the widespread integration and accessibility of NGS in the initial workup of cytopenic patients. Updated WHO-HAEM5 and ICC guidelines as well as the new IPSS-M place an emphasis on molecular data into the diagnosis, classification, and prognostication of MDS, compared to previous tools that were based more heavily on clinical findings, morphology, or cytogenetics only.[1,2,34]

Novel therapeutic approaches are needed to improve outcomes in patients with MDS with multi-hit *TP53* mutations. Further research is needed to understand the optimal management of TP53-mutated patients with MDS. The development of new therapies that target *TP53* mutations may provide hope for improved outcomes in this high-risk patient population. Additionally, ongoing efforts to identify and characterize other genetic and epigenetic alterations that contribute to the pathogenesis of MDS may lead to more personalized approaches to patient care in the future.

CLINICS CARE POINTS

- TP53-mutated MDS frequently is associate with a complex karyotype and represents a group of patients with an adverse prognosis.
- Updated WHO-HAEM5 and ICC classification schemes for 2022 place a significant emphasis on genetically defined disease. Specifically, there are strict criteria defining the molecular profile of TP53-mutated MDS, while there is more flexibility with the morphologic blast count.
- The incorporation of NGS into routine MDS evaluations has revolutionized disease diagnosis, shaped prognosis, and drives personalized therapy.

FUNDING AND CONFLICTS OF INTEREST

The authors report no relevant conflicts of interest, financial or otherwise.

REFERENCES

1. Arber DA, Orazi A, Hasserjian RP, et al. International consensus classification of myeloid neoplasms and acute leukemias: integrating morphologic, clinical, and genomic data. Blood 2022;140(11):1200–28.
2. Khoury JD, Solary E, Abla O, et al. The 5th edition of the World Health organization classification of haematolymphoid tumours: myeloid and histiocytic/dendritic neoplasms. Leukemia 2022;36(7):1703–19.
3. Malcovati L, Hellstrom-Lindberg E, Bowen D, et al. Diagnosis and treatment of primary myelodysplastic syndromes in adults: recommendations from the European LeukemiaNet. Blood 2013;122:2943–64.
4. Papaemmanuil E, Gerstung M, Malcovati L, et al. Clinical and biological implications of driver mutations in myelodysplastic syndromes. Blood 2013;122: 3616–27.
5. Vousden KH, Prives C. Blinded by the light: the growing complexity of p53. Cell 2009;137(3):413–31.
6. Bykov VJN, Eriksson SE, Bianchi J, et al. Targeting mutant p53 for efficient cancer therapy. Nat Rev Cancer 2018;18(2):89–102.
7. Bode AM, Dong Z. Post-translational modification of p53 in tumorigenesis. Nat Rev Cancer 2004;4(10):793–805.
8. Levine AJ. p53: 800 million years of evolution and 40 years of discovery. Nat Rev Cancer 2020;20471–80.
9. Pant V, Quintás-Cardama A, Lozano G. The p53 pathway in hematopoiesis: lessons from mouse models, implications for humans. Blood 2012;120:5118–27.
10. Jaiswal S, Fontanillas P, Flannick J, et al. Age-related clonal hematopoiesis associated with adverse outcomes. N Engl J Med 2014;371:2488–98.
11. Liu Y, Elf SE, Miyata Y, et al. p53 regulates hematopoietic stem cell quiescence. Cell Stem Cell 2009;4(1):37–48.
12. Huang J. Current developments of targeting the p53 signaling pathway for cancer treatment. Pharmacol Ther 2021;220:107720.
13. Bernard E, Nannya Y, Hasserjian RP, et al. Implications of *TP53* allelic state for genome stability, clinical presentation and outcomes in myelodysplastic syndromes. Nat Med 2020;26:1549–56.
14. Lindsley RC, Saber W, Mar BG, et al. Prognostic mutations in myelodysplastic syndrome after stem cell transplantation. N Engl J Med 2017;376:536–47.
15. Ok CY, Patel KP, Garcia-Manero G, et al. *TP53* mutation characteristics in therapy-related myelodysplastic syndromes and acute myeloid leukemia is similar to de novo diseases. J Hematol Oncol 2015;8:45.
16. Haase D, Stevenson KE, Neuberg D, et al. *TP53* mutation status divides myelodysplastic syndromes with complex karyotypes into distinct prognostic subgroups. Leukemia 2019;33(7):1747–58.
17. Weinberg OK, Siddon A, Madanat YF, et al. *TP53* mutation defines a unique subgroup within complex karyotype de novo and therapy-related MDS/AML. Blood Adv 2022;6(9):2847–53.
18. Stengel A, Kern W, Haferlach T, et al. The impact of *TP53* mutations and *TP53* deletions on survival varies between AML, ALL, MDS and CLL: an analysis of 3307 cases. Leukemia 2017;31(3):705–11.

19. Wong TN, Ramsingh G, Young AL, et al. Role of *TP53* mutations in the origin and evolution of therapy-related acute myeloid leukaemia. Nature 2015;518(7540): 552-5.
20. Lai JL, Preudhomme C, Zandecki M, et al. Myelodysplastic syndromes and acute myeloid leukemia with 17p deletion. An entity characterized by specific dysgranulopoïesis and a high incidence of P53 mutations. Leukemia 1995;9(3):370-81.
21. Sabapathy K, Lane DP. Therapeutic targeting of p53: all mutants are equal, but some mutants are more equal than others. Nat Rev Clin Oncol 2018;15(1):13-30.
22. Klimovich B, Merle N, Neumann M, et al. p53 partial loss-of-function mutations sensitize to chemotherapy. Oncogene 2022;41(7):1011-23.
23. Boettcher S, Miller PG, Sharma R, et al. A dominant-negative effect drives selection of *TP53* missense mutations in myeloid malignancies. Science 2019; 365(6453):599-604.
24. Christiansen DH, Andersen MK, Pedersen-Bjergaard J. Mutations with loss of heterozygosity of p53 are common in therapy-related myelodysplasia and acute myeloid leukemia after exposure to alkylating agents and significantly associated with deletion or loss of 5q, a complex karyotype, and a poor prognosis. J Clin Oncol 2001;19(5):1405-13.
25. Swerdlow SH, Campo E, Harris NL, et al. WHO classification of tumours of haematopoietic and lymphoid tissues. 4th ed. Lyon, France: IARC; 2017.
26. Grob T, Al Hinai ASA, Sanders MA, et al. Molecular characterization of mutant *TP53* acute myeloid leukemia and high-risk myelodysplastic syndrome. Blood 2022;139:2347-54.
27. Duncavage EJ, Bagg A, Hasserjian RP, et al. Genomic profiling for clinical decision making in myeloid neoplasms and acute leukemia. Blood 2022;140(21): 2228-47.
28. Smith TA, Whelan J, Parry PJ. Detection of single-base mutations in a mixed population of cells: a comparison of SSCP and direct sequencing. Genet Anal Tech Appl 1992;9(5-6):143-5.
29. Merlat A, Lai JL, Sterkers Y, et al. Therapy-related myelodysplastic syndrome and acute myeloid leukemia with 17p deletion. A report on 25 cases. Leukemia 1999; 13(2):250-7.
30. Greenberg PL, Stone RM, Al-Kali A, et al. NCCN guidelines® insights: myelodysplastic syndromes, version 3.2022. J Natl Compr Cancer Netw 2022;20(2): 106-17.
31. Greenberg PL, Tuechler H, Schanz J, et al. Revised international prognostic scoring system for myelodysplastic syndromes. Blood 2012;120(12):2454-65.
32. DeZern AE. Lower risk but high risk. Hematology Am Soc Hematol Educ Program 2021;2021(1):428-34.
33. Haferlach T, Nagata Y, Grossman V, et al. Landscape of genetic lesions in 944 patients with myelodysplastic syndromes. Leukemia 2014;28(2):241-7.
34. Bernard E, Tuechler H, Greenberg PL, et al. Molecular international pognostic scoring system for myelodyplastic syndromes. NEJM Evid 2022;1(7).
35. Kewan T, Bahaj W, Durmaz A, et al. Validation of the molecular international prognostic scoring system in patients with myelodysplastic syndromes. Blood 2023; 141(14):1768-72.

Germline Predisposition to Myeloid Neoplasms

Diagnostic Concepts and Classifications

Ifeyinwa E. Obiorah, MD, PhD[a], Kalpana D. Upadhyaya, PhD[b],
Katherine R. Calvo, MD, PhD[b,c],*

KEYWORDS

- Germline predisposition • MDS • AML • DDX41 • RUNX1 • GATA2 • SAMD9L
- CEBPA

KEY POINTS

- Identification of myeloid malignancies with germline predisposition is critical for proper patient care, genetic counseling, informing donor selection for hematopoietic stem cell transplantation and conditioning regimens.
- In general, myeloid neoplasms with germline predisposition develop at a younger age than sporadic neoplasms; however, some germline mutations predispose to malignancy that develops in older patients (eg, *DDX41*).
- Germline mutations may be inherited and present in multiple family members or *de novo* and found in the patient and not in parents or siblings (ie, no family history).
- Germline mutations should be considered in patients diagnosed with a myeloid neoplasm:
  - At a young age (less than 40 years).
  - With a prior history of cancer.
  - If there is a family history of hematologic neoplasms, other cancers, or bone marrow failure.
  - If there is a preceding history of thrombocytopenia, bone marrow failure, immunodeficiency, warts, lymphedema, early graying of hair, pulmonary/hepatic fibrosis, or other syndromic features associated with specific germline mutations.

INTRODUCTION

Inherited hematologic neoplasms are rare underdiagnosed entities that have gained recognition due to increased sequencing and detection of germline variants associated with myelodysplastic syndrome (MDS) and acute myeloid leukemia (AML).

[a] Department of Pathology, Division of Hematopathology, University of Virginia Health, Charlottesville, VA, USA; [b] Hematology Section, Department of Laboratory Medicine, Clinical Center, National Institutes of Health, Bethesda, MD, USA; [c] Myeloid Malignancies Program, National Institutes of Health, Bethesda, MD, USA
* Corresponding author. Hematology Section, Department of Laboratory Medicine, National Institutes of Health Clinical Center, Bethesda, MD 20892-1508.
E-mail address: calvok@mail.nih.gov

Clin Lab Med 43 (2023) 615–638
https://doi.org/10.1016/j.cll.2023.06.004
0272-2712/23/Published by Elsevier Inc.
labmed.theclinics.com

Hereditary hematologic malignancies are often diagnosed based on personal or family history of multiple cancers or hematopoietic neoplasms at early age in comparison to the general population, thrombocytopenia and platelet associated disorders, immunodeficiency, and/or phenotypic signs of genetic cancer syndromes.[1] Failure to recognize germline predisposition often results from lack of awareness of the characteristic features of germline-related myeloid neoplasms by the treating physician or pathologist, or absence of filters to discriminate between somatic and germline variants during molecular profiling. Consequently, the identification of patients who might benefit from genetic mutational testing is important for surveillance for disease progression and therapeutic management including donor selection for hematopoietic stem cell transplantation (HSCT), and genetic counseling. Multiple studies have shown that patients with germline mutations and hematologic malignancy who were inadvertently transplanted using a healthy related donor that harbored the same germline mutation resulted in donor-derived MDS/AML, failed engraftment, fatal infections, or other avoidable negative outcomes[2–5]

Germline mutations may be inherited from parents in an autosomal dominant, recessive, or X-linked pattern. De novo germline mutations are present in the patient and not present in either parent. De novo germline mutations may arise in a sperm, ova, or in the fertilized egg during embryogenesis, and can be passed on to offspring.[6] Many germline mutations are detected in blood or bone marrow samples on next generation sequencing (NGS) panels designed to detect somatic mutations in cancer. In these instances, the germline mutation often has a high variant allele frequency (VAF) of 30% to 60%[7] which can also be seen in somatic mutations in hematopoietic tumor cells. Therefore, it is essential to confirm potential germline mutations with specialized germline testing on a germline tissue sample such as DNA from skin fibroblast culture. Germline mutations can also be strongly suggested by repeat NGS testing post-treatment where the VAF of somatic mutation will be lower after treatment whereas the germline mutation VAF remains unchanged. If the same potential germline mutation is found in other family members, this supports the germline nature of the mutation. Importantly, patients may have mutations in non-coding regions of the gene that can be missed by whole exome sequencing and NGS targeted panels that do not cover non-coding regions. Large deletions/insertions may also be missed by NGS testing.

Myeloid-related neoplasms are well established in the setting of inherited cancer syndromes and often present in childhood/young adulthood. By contrast, not all family members with an inherited mutation has clinical manifestations due to variable penetrance and expressivity. Thus, some individuals may be normal or clinical disease may manifest in older adulthood with specific signs and symptoms often differing among affected individuals in the same family. Myeloid neoplasms with germline predisposition were introduced as a distinct category in the revised 2017 4th edition of the WHO Classification of Tumors of Haematopoietic and Lymphoid Tissues.[8] This underscored the importance of the recognition of these disorders during diagnostic workup in patients with myeloid or lymphoid tumors. Until recently in the absence of syndromic features, CEBPA, DDX41, RUNX1, ANKRD26, ETV6, and GATA2 were among the more commonly reported genes with germline mutations known to cause familial MDS/AML. At the same time, there is a growing list of genes identified in recent years that has been included in this category by the new ICC classification[9] and the 2022 WHO 5th edition classification[10] such as TP53, SAMD9, and SAMD9L.

In this review, we will address both the previous and recently described predisposition genes in familial AML and MDS (**Table 1**). We will discuss the key findings of the clinical and genetic spectrum and emphasize the diagnostic approach by

Table 1
Hematologic neoplasms with germline predisposition

Familial Syndrome	Gene	Inheritance	Pathogenic Mechanism	Hematologic Malignancy	Non-hematologic Malignancy	Clinical Presentation	Recurrent Somatic Alterations
Hematologic neoplasms with germline predisposition without a constitutional disorder affecting multiple organ systems							
Myeloid neoplasms with germline CEBPA mutation	CEBPA	Autosomal dominant	Altered transcription factor regulation	AML	None reported	Blasts with frequent auer rods and CD7 expression on and normal karyotype	Mutation in the second CEBPA allele
Myeloid or lymphoid neoplasms with germline DDX41 mutation	DDX41	Autosomal dominant	Unknown but genetic mutations that encode RNA splicing-related factors implicated	MDS and AML. Less commonly, follicular lymphoma, Hodgkin lymphoma and multiple myeloma	None reported	Age of onset of myeloid neoplasms is often in adulthood. Hypocellular BM, often with prominent dyserythropoiesis and normal karyotypes	Mutation in the second DDX41 allele Additional CHIP mutations such as ASXLI, DNMT3A, TET2, TP53
Myeloid or lymphoid neoplasms with germline TP53 mutation	TP53	Autosomal dominant	Altered DNA binding/ repair and transactivation of P53-responsive genes	Hypodiploid B lymphoblastic leukemia/lymphoma. Less frequently AML and therapy-related myeloid neoplasms including MDS	Solid tumors, including osteosarcomas, adrenocortical carcinomas, CNS tumors, and soft tissue sarcomas, are common	Congenital anomalies	Mutation in the second TP53 allele Complex karyotype
Hematologic neoplasms with germline predisposition associated with a constitutional platelet disorder							
Myeloid or lymphoid neoplasms with germline RUNX1 mutation	RUNX1	Autosomal dominant	Altered transcription factor function	AML and MDS, less frequently CMML, T-ALL, and more rarely B-cell malignancies	None reported	Thrombocytopenia, platelet defects, bleeding tendency. Hypocellular marrow and abnormal megakaryopoiesis. Pediatric or adult onset of MN	Mutation in the second RUNX1 allele. Additional somatic mutations in GATA2, CBL, DNMT3A, KRAS, FLT3, as well as monosomy 7

(continued on next page)

Table 1
(continued)

Familial Syndrome	Gene	Inheritance	Pathogenic Mechanism	Hematologic Malignancy	Non-hematologic Malignancy	Clinical Presentation	Recurrent Somatic Alterations
Myeloid neoplasms with germline ANKRD26 mutation	ANKRD26	Autosomal dominant	Abnormal signaling through the MPL pathway and impaired proplatelet formation	AML and MDS, less frequently CML, CMML, and CLL	None reported	Thrombocytopenia, platelet defects, bleeding tendency. Hypocellular marrow and abnormal megakaryopoiesis. Adult onset of MN	
Myeloid or lymphoid neoplasms with germline ETV6 mutation	ETV6	Autosomal dominant	Altered DNA binding, abnormal subcellular localization, reduced transcriptional repression and impaired hematopoiesis	B lymphoblastic leukemia (most common), MDS, AML, CMML, and myeloma	Colorectal carcinoma and breast cancer	Thrombocytopenia, normal platelet size, bleeding tendency. Hypocellular marrow and abnormal megakaryopoiesis. Dyserythropoiesis may be prominent	
Hematologic neoplasms with germline predisposition associated with a constitutional disorder affecting multiple organ systems							
Myeloid neoplasms with germline GATA2 mutation	GATA2	Autosomal dominant	Altered transcription factor function	MDS, AML, CMML	Solid tumors	Immunodeficiency, lymphedema, warts, and other multiple phenotypes. Adolescent and young adult onset of MN are common	ASXL1, STAG2, SETBP1, RUNX1, IKZF1, PTPN11, CRLF2, monosomy 7, trisomy 8
Myeloid neoplasms with germline SAMD9 mutation	SAMD9	Autosomal dominant	Abnormal cellular proliferation pathways	MDS, AML with monosomy 7	N/A	MIRAGE (Myelodysplasia (monosomy 7), Infections, Restriction of growth, Adrenal hypoplasia, Genital phenotypes and Enteropathy) syndrome. Revertant somatic mosaicism can occur	ASXL1, RUNX1, SETBP1, KRAS, PTPN11, CBL, EZH2, ETV6, BRAF, RAD21

Myeloid neoplasms with germline SAMD9L mutation	SAMD9L	Autosomal dominant	Abnormal cellular proliferation pathways	MDS, AML with monosomy 7	N/A	Ataxia-pancytopenia (AP) syndrome. cerebellar ataxia, variable cytopenias, marrow failure) Revertant somatic mosaicism can occur	ASXL1, RUNX1, SETBP1, KRAS, PTPN11, CBL, EZH2 ETV6, BRAF, RAD21
Myeloid neoplasms associated with bone marrow failure syndromes							
Fanconi anemia	FANC genes	Autosomal recessive (most common, 22 genes FANCB is X-linked recessive FANCR is autosomal dominant)	Defects of DNA repair and FA pathway causing chromosomal instability and cellular hypersensitivity to interstrand DNA crosslinking agents	MDS and AML	Squamous cell carcinoma of the skin, head and neck, and vulva. Liver tumors	Congenital anomalies, Aplastic anemia. Childhood onset of MN	Gain of 3q, Gain of 1q, deletion 7q, monosomy 7, complex, RUNX1
Shwachman–Diamond syndrome	SBDS (most common) DNAJC21, EFL1, SRP54	Autosomal recessive	Impaired ribosome assembly	MDS and AML	Rare	Multisystem disease, Hypocellular marrow with myeloid hypoplasia and mild dyspoieisis Common cytogenetic abnormalities include 20q deletion and isochromome 7q (not associated with high risk of progression to MDS/AML	TP53 (~50% of cases with SBDS germline mutation), monosomy 7/del7q Biallelic TP53 mutations in MN
Telomere biology disorders including dyskeratosis congenita	DKC1, TERT, TERC, TINF2, ACD, POT1, RTEL1, NAF1, STN1, WRAP53, NOP10, NHP2	AD, AR, and X linked	Telomere maintenance alteration leading to chromosome instability and apoptosis	MDS and AML	High risk of solid tumors such as squamous cell carcinoma	Cytopenias red cell macrocytosis, aplastic anemia nail dystrophy, abnormal skin and pigmentation, oral leukoplakia, early hair graying, pulmonary fibrosis, hepatic fibrosis	Monosomy 7 Somatic mutations are uncommon

(continued on next page)

Table 1
(continued)

Familial Syndrome	Gene	Inheritance	Pathogenic Mechanism	Hematologic Malignancy	Non-hematologic Malignancy	Clinical Presentation	Recurrent Somatic Alterations
Severe congenital neutropenia	ELANE(most common) CSF3R, GFI1, CXCR2, G6PC3 HAX1 WAS	Autosomal dominance (ELANE, CSF3R and GFI1), autosomal recessive (CXCR2, HAX1, and G6PC3) or X-linked (WAS) patterns	Missense mutations inducing an abnormal survival of bone marrow progenitor cells	MDS and AML	Less frequent, including HPV associated carcinomas	Severe opportunistic infections in neonatal period. Bone marrow evaluation reveals a maturation arrest at the level of promyelocytes. Eosinophilia and monocytosis may be present	Monosomy 7, RUNX1, CSF3R
Diamond-Blackfan anemia	RPS19, RPS17, RPS24, RPL35 A RPL5, RPL11, RPL15, RPL26 RPS7, RPS26, RPS10, RPS29	Autosomal dominant		MDS and AML	Solid tumors	Congenital anomalies, severe macrocytic anemia in infancy, reticulocytopenia and elevated erythrocyte adenosine deaminase BM with erythroid hypoplasia and immature erythroid precursors with maturation arrest	
Juvenile myelomonocytic leukemia associated with neurofibromatosis	NF1	Autosomal dominance	Disruption of the RAS pathway signaling	Childhood JMML, AML, ALL later in life	Solid tumors particularly of the nervous system	Multiple café au lait spots, axillary and inguinal freckling, cutaneous neurofibromas, iris Lisch nodules, and choroidal freckling are frequent	Acquired uniparental disomy of the mutated allele and additional RAS pathway mutations

Juvenile myelomonocytic leukemia associated with Noonan-syndrome-like disorder	PTPN11, NRAS, KRAS	Autosomal dominance	Disruption of the RAS pathway signaling	Childhood JMML, ALL later in life	Solid tumors	Noonan syndrome-like developmental anomalies with variable expressivity	Acquired uniparental disomy of the mutated allele and additional RAS pathway mutations
Myeloid or lymphoid neoplasms associated with Down syndrome	Trisomy 21	N/A	Abnormal fetal hematopoiesis with an acquired mutation in *GATA1*	Transient abnormal myelopoiesis AML(acute megakaryoblastic Leukemia, 50%), B-ALL	Low risk of solid tumors	Multiple development Anomalies, childhood onset of MN	Secondary somatic mutations for example, *STAG2, SMC1/3, CTCF, KANSL1, EZH2,* and *SUZ12, MPL, KIT*

integrating clinical history, bone marrow morphology, cytogenetics, and molecular methods.

HEMATOLOGIC NEOPLASMS WITH GERMLINE PREDISPOSITION WITHOUT A CONSTITUTIONAL DISORDER AFFECTING MULTIPLE ORGAN SYSTEMS

Myeloid Neoplasms with Germline CEBPA Mutation

The transcription factor CCAAT/enhancer binding protein-α (CEBPA), a transcription factor, is encoded on chromosome 19q13.1 and is crucial for normal myeloid differentiation.[11] Mutations can be subdivided into the N-terminal frame-shift mutations, which result in premature truncation of the full-length 42 kDa form while enhancing the production of the alternate dominant-negative 30 kDa form, and the less frequent C-terminal inframe insertions/deletions that disrupt DNA binding and homo- and heterodimerization with other CEBP family members.[12] Hence, the AML induced by the germline CEBPA mutation is an autosomal dominant inherited disorder, associated with biallelic inactivation of the gene.[8] The germline CEBPA mutations are mostly clustered within the N-terminal and show complete or near complete penetrance, when compared with the C terminal mutations, which demonstrate a lower penetrance for AML development.[13,14] Twana and colleagues[14] performed the first comprehensive study of familial CEBPA mutated cases and demonstrated that majority of the AML cases frequently present in children and young adults with a median age of 24.5 years. Unlike other many other AML predisposition syndromes, germline CEBPA mutations are associated with sudden onset of disease, without a preceding MDS or cytopenic phase. The development of AML is typically associated with an acquired somatic mutation as a second event.[14,15] Histologic features are similar to that observed with somatic CEBPA associated AML with frequent Auer rods, CD7 expression on the blasts and normal karyotype. In addition, these patients with familial CEBPA mutations show favorable long-term overall survival (10 year overall survival, 67%). In contrast to CEBPA mutations in sporadic AML, patients with relapses in familial CEBPA AML, following chemotherapy, developed new clones including new somatic CEBPA mutations. Thus, this may represent the development of a second primary AML rather than true disease recurrence. Perhaps a better strategy for treatment for these patients should include allogeneic stem cell transplantation in first remission to prevent subsequent development of new AML clones.

Myeloid or Lymphoid Neoplasms with Germline DDX41 Mutation

The DEAD-box helicase 41 (DDX41) gene, located on chromosome 5q35, encodes a DEAD-box type RNA helicase and plays important roles in biological processes related to RNA metabolism.[16] Because the RNA helicase has multiple cellular functions, the exact oncogenic mechanism of DDX41 involvement in leukemogenesis remains unclear. However, the enzyme has been implicated in the regulation of RNA splicing. Genetic mutations that encode RNA splicing-related factors implicated in myeloid malignancies are involved in the recognition and determination of 3′ splice sites. In contrast, the nature of the RNA splicing alterations in DDX41 related cases are specific to each mutated splicing factor, and is likely incorporated into the C complex of the spliceosome, which may result in a distinct phenotype.[17] Pathogenesis is proposed to occur in a stepwise manner. Significant number of familial cases harbors heterozygous germline DDX41 variants, which may result in normal or mildly impaired hematopoiesis such as cytopenias and macrocytosis.[18] A significant number of cases are associated with acquisition of somatic DDX41 mutations, usually in older age, resulting in biallelic aberration and development of overt myeloid neoplasm

(Fig. 1).[18,19] Patients with germline *DDX1* mutations frequency present with late onset development of MDS and AML, and a high frequency of normal karyotypes. The bone marrow of DDX41 germline MDS cases are typically hypocellular, often with prominent dyserythropoiesis. Lymphoid neoplasms have been less frequently described in familial *DDX41* mutated patients. In addition to myeloid malignancies, Lewinsohn and colleagues[19] detected follicular lymphoma, Hodgkin lymphoma and multiple myeloma in a subset of patients with germline *DDX41* mutations.

Myeloid or Lymphoid Neoplasms with Germline TP53 Mutation

The *TP53* tumor suppressor gene regulates critical processes, such as apoptosis, cell cycle arrest, DNA repair, senescence, and cellular metabolism.[20] Germline mutation of TP53 results in Li-Fraumeni syndrome (LFS), a rare autosomal dominant syndrome.[21] The majority of familial *TP53* mutations are missense mutations that prevent DNA binding and transactivation of *P53*-responsive genes.[20] In childhood, the tumor spectrum of LFS is characterized by osteosarcomas, adrenocortical carcinomas, central nervous system (CNS) tumors, and soft tissue sarcomas.[22] Only a small proportion of these patients develop hematologic malignancies. The most commonly reported leukemia in germline *TP53* mutations is hypodiploid B lymphoblastic leukemia/lymphoma,[23] and to a lesser extent, AML and therapy-related myeloid neoplasms including MDS.[23,24] Hypodiploid ALL can exist in either near haploidy or low

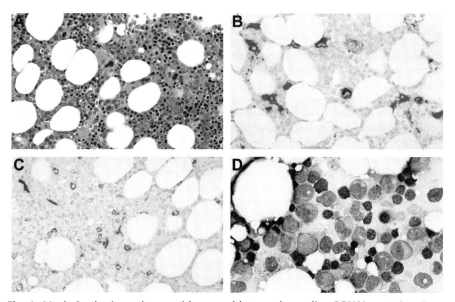

Fig. 1. Myelodysplastic syndrome with excess blasts and germline DDX41 mutation. Bone marrow from a male in his 60s with a family history of AML in one sibling. (*A*) Normocellular marrow with atypical megakaryocytes and erythroid predominance, left shift in myeloid maturation (H&E, 500×). (*B*) CD61 immunostain shows multiple small dysplastic megakaryocytes (500×). (*C*) CD34 demonstrates increased positive cells consistent with myeloblasts (7%) identified by flow cytometry analysis that were positive for CD34, CD13, HLA-DR, with atypical expression of CD7 and lack of CD38 (not shown) (500×). (*D*) Aspirate smear with increased blasts and left shift in myeloid maturation (WG stain, 1000×). Cytogenetics revealed a normal karyotype. NGS analysis showed 2 DDX41 mutations, one germline (confirmed sequencing cultured fibroblasts from skin biopsy) and the other somatic.

hypodiploid states. The low hypodiploid ALL are associated with distinct additional somatic mutations and deletions, commonly affecting the *IKZF2, CDKN2A,* and *CDKN2B* genes.[24] In addition, the low hypodiploid, but not near haploid ALL has near-universal mutation of *TP53*,[25] with nearly half having germline *TP53* mutations.[23] Thus, detection of low hypodiploidy in pediatric ALL should raise the suspicion of a germline *TP53* variant.

HEMATOLOGIC NEOPLASMS WITH GERMLINE PREDISPOSITION ASSOCIATED WITH A CONSTITUTIONAL PLATELET DISORDER

Myeloid or Lymphoid Neoplasms with Germline RUNX1 Mutation

Germline heterozygous mutations in *RUNX1* (chromosome 21q22), with an autosomal dominant inheritance pattern, were first reported in 1999[26] in patients with a familial platelet disorder (FPD) and propensity to develop AML. Germline mutations include insertions, deletions, missense, nonsense, and frameshift mutations in the *RUNX1* gene.[27] *RUNX1* (also known as *CBFA2*) encodes the DNA-binding subunit of the core-binding factor transcription complex that is necessary for normal hematopoiesis. Heterozygous germline mutations in *RUNX1* are present in patients with FPD and carriers show a variation of clinical manifestations ranging from being asymptomatic to presenting with thrombocytopenia, platelet defects, bleeding tendencies, or development of a hematologic malignancy. The lifetime risk of MDS/AML is estimated at approximately 40% with onset at an average age of 34 (range 6–72 years).[28] *In vitro* studies have shown that megakaryocytes in RUNX1 FPD have low ploidy and impaired proplatelet formation.[29] The bone marrow of patients with isolated thrombocytopenia with otherwise normal peripheral blood counts is typically normocellular or hypocellular with evidence of dysmegakaryopoiesis composed of small mono- or hypolobated megakaryocytes with impaired maturation (**Fig. 2**). Pathologists are cautioned not to overdiagnose MDS in RUNX1 FDP patients with dysmegakaropoiesis in the setting of isolated thrombocytopenia. Progression to overt MDS is associated with additional cytopenias, hypercellularity, multilineage dysplasia (with erythroid and/or myeloid dysplasia in addition to dysmegakaryopoiesis), increased blasts, and/or additional acquired cytogenetic/molecular abnormalities[30] (**Fig. 3**). The most common malignancies are AML and MDS and to a lesser extent; chronic myelomonocytic leukemia (CMML), T lymphoblastic leukemia/lymphoma, B lymphoblastic leukemia, and rarely B-cell lymphoma. Myeloid tumors in these patients show enrichment for somatic mutations affecting the second *RUNX1* allele and *GATA2* and less commonly, *CBL, DNMT3A, KRAS,* and *FLT3*.[27,31]

Myeloid Neoplasms with Germline ANKRD26 Mutation

Thrombocytopenia 2 is an autosomal dominant disease, characterized by ankyrin repeat domain 26 (ANKRD26) germline mutation usually in the 5' untranslated region[32] located on chromosome band 10p12.1. Both RUNX1 and FLI1 transcription factors bind to the 5' UTR of the *ANKRD26* gene leading to repression of gene transcription. The germline mutations are gain of function resulting in abnormal signaling through the *MPL* pathway and impaired proplatelet formation by megakaryocytes.[33] Patients with familial *ANKRD26* mutations often present with moderate thrombocytopenia, a deficiency of platelet α-granules, normal *in vitro* platelet aggregation, normal mean platelet volume, and a predisposition to MDS and AML.[34] Thrombopoietin levels are elevated in these patients and bleeding tendencies are mild. Similar to RUNX1 FPD, bone marrow morphologic findings at baseline are characterized by prominent megakaryocytic atypia including small hypolobated forms and micromegakaryocytes that

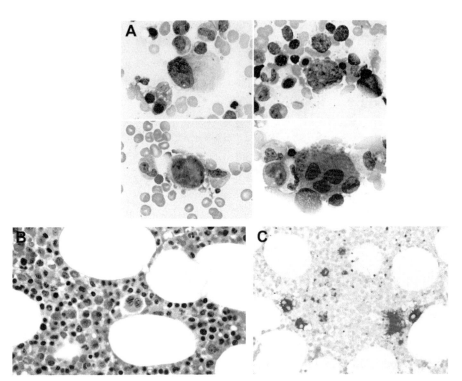

Fig. 2. Dysmegakaryopoiesis in baseline bone marrows of patients with RUNX1 familial platelet disorder (FPD) and isolated thrombocytopenia, not representing MDS. (*A*) Composite of abnormal megakaryocytes that can be seen in RUNX1 FPD patients who do not have MDS, demonstrating abnormal impaired megakaryopoiesis including mononuclear forms with eccentric nuclei and presence of cytoplasm, abnormal small forms with hypolobated nuclei and minimal scant cytoplasm with surface blebbing, and forms with separated nuclear lobes (aspirates, WG stain, 1000×). (*B*) Core biopsy showing abnormal small megakaryocyte with appearance of separated nuclear lobes (H&E, 500×). (*C*) CD61 immunohistochemistry stain on core biopsy showing a subset of very small mononuclear megakaryocytes (500×).

can lead to a misdiagnosis of MDS.[35] The risk of developing myeloid neoplasms is approximately 30 times greater than the general population. Although germline *ANKRD26* mutations are associated with mostly MDS and AML, a small number of patients with chronic myeloid leukemia (CML), CMML, and chronic lymphocytic leukemia (CLL) have been reported.[36]

Myeloid or Lymphoid Neoplasms with Germline ETV6 Mutation

Germline heterozygous mutations in ETS variant transcription factor 6 (*ETV6*) (chromosome 12p13), with an autosomal dominant inheritance pattern, was first described as a translocation partner of PDGFB in CMML in 1994.[37] *ETV6* is essential in early embryonic development and adult hematopoiesis. Germline mutations involving the *ETV6* gene were first report in 2015 in families with thrombocytopenia and predisposition to hematologic malignancy.[38–40] The germline mutations are often missense mutations, which disrupt DNA binding, alter subcellular localization, and reduce transcriptional repression in a dominant-negative fashion thereby impairing hematopoiesis.[41] The common phenotype of carriers of *ETV6* mutations is mild-to-moderate

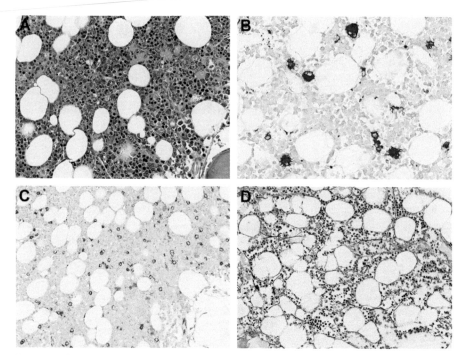

Fig. 3. Myelodysplastic syndrome with excess blasts and germline mutation in RUNX1 FPD. (*A*) Mildly hypocellular bone marrow core biopsy from a male in his 30s with thrombocytopenia and mild anemia (500×). (*B*) CD61 immunostain shows multiple small dysplastic megakaryocytes (500×), (*C*) CD34 shows increased positive cells consistent with myeloblasts (8%) identified by flow cytometry analysis showing an abnormal immunophenotype lacking CD38 (not shown) (500×). (*D*) Reticulin stain showing increased reticulin fibrosis (500×); aspirate smear was paucicellular. Cytogenetic analysis revealed a normal karyotype.

thrombocytopenia, with normal-sized platelets and mild-to-moderate bleeding tendency. Bone marrow biopsies often exhibit increased small hypolobated megakaryocytes and mild degrees of dyserythropoiesis. Germline *ETV6* mutations predispose to both myeloid and lymphoid tumors. Leukemia is estimated to occur in approximately 30% of carriers, with B precursor acute lymphoblastic leukemia (B-ALL) being most frequent.[39] However, MDS, AML, CMML, and plasma cell myeloma have also been reported. There is also familial predisposition for solid tumors including colorectal adenocarcinoma.

Germline mutations in *ETV6, RUNX1,* or *ANKRD26* should be considered in patients with thrombocytopenia, bone marrows with isolated dysmegakaryopoiesis and a family history of bleeding and/or hematologic malignancies. Notably, the dysmegakaryopoiesis observed does not necessarily equate to MDS. Transformation to MDS is associated with additional cytopenias, multilineage dysplasia, increased blasts, and/or cytogenetic abnormalities.

HEMATOLOGIC NEOPLASMS WITH GERMLINE PREDISPOSITION ASSOCIATED WITH A CONSTITUTIONAL DISORDER AFFECTING MULTIPLE ORGAN SYSTEMS
Myeloid Neoplasms with Germline GATA2 Mutation

Germline *GATA2* gene mutations were originally reported in 2011 as 4 separate syndromes with predisposition to MDS/AML including MonoMac syndrome (characterized by monocytopenia and mycobacterium avium complex infections),[42] dendritic cell, monocyte, B, and natural killer (NK) lymphoid (DCML) deficiency,[43] familial MDS/AML,[44] and Emberger syndrome (characterized by lymphedema, warts, and MDS/AML predisposition).[45] These disorders with overlapping features were subsequently recognized as a single genetic disorder with variable manifestations now called GATA2 deficiency.[46] GATA2 is located on chromosome 3q21.3, contains 7 exons, and encodes a zinc-finger transcription factor that is essential for regulating hematopoiesis, autoimmunity, and inflammation.[47] Germline mutations are transmitted with autosomal dominant inheritance and involve both coding and noncoding regions, resulting in haploinsufficiency.[48] The clinical manifestations of GATA2 deficiency are heterogeneous and result in a combination of cytopenias, immunodeficiency, and increased risk of infections such as nontuberculous mycobacterial infections, severe viral including disseminated warts, and invasive fungal infections. The resultant effect includes bone marrow stress, hypocellularity, bone marrow failure, and predisposition to MDS.[43] Although a small subset of cases present with AML, many patients present with an initial hypoplastic marrow with or without overt MDS and have a high risk of evolution to AML or CMML[49] (Fig. 4). Other manifestations of germline GATA2 mutations include lymphedema, sensorineural hearing loss, and pulmonary alveolar proteinosis. GATA2 mutations were also identified in a small number of cases of congenital neutropenia and aplastic anemia.[50] Approximately 75% of GATA2 mutation carriers develop myeloid neoplasms at an estimated median age of 20 years.[51] Bone marrow examination of GATA2 deficiency often demonstrates a hypocellular marrow with varying degrees of dysplasia, and can overlap morphologically with aplastic anemia. Dysmegakaryopoiesis is the most prominent dysplasia and increased reticulin fibrosis may be present. Flow cytometry analysis of the bone marrow aspirate can be helpful in differentiating GATA2 deficiency from idiopathic/immune aplastic anemia as GATA2 deficiency typically shows disproportionate loss of monocytes, dendritic cells, NK cells, and precursor B cells, which are typically present in aplastic anemia.[50] Germline GATA2 mutations are present in up to 7% of pediatric MDS patients overall, and up to 75% of adolescents with MDS and monosomy 7 and majority meet the criteria for refractory anemia of childhood (RCC).[52] A subset of bone marrows in GATA2 patients with cytopenias and infections show no overt dysplasia and normal karyotype and are termed bone marrow and immunodeficiency disorder with germline GATA2 mutation.[53] These GATA2 patients must be carefully monitored as the risk for transformation to overt MDS/AML is high. Notably, up to 20% of patients harbor germline GATA2 mutations in an intronic enhancer element that may be missed on whole exome sequencing or NGS panels that do not cover this region.[54]

Myeloid Neoplasms with Germline SAMD9 or SAMD9L Mutation

Sterile alpha motif domain-containing protein 9 (SAMD9) and the paralog gene SAMD9-like (SAMD9L) are located alongside each other on chromosome 7q21. Germline mutations in SAMD9 were first reported as MIRAGE (Myelodysplasia (monosomy 7), Infections, and Restriction of growth, Adrenal hypoplasia, Genital phenotypes and Enteropathy) syndrome in 2016.[55] A parallel study[56] detected missense mutations in SAMD9L in ataxia-pancytopenia (AP) syndrome. AP is characterized by cerebellar ataxia, variable cytopenias, marrow failure, and MDS/AML, sometimes associated with monosomy 7. Both studies exhibited a common phenotype of early onset MDS with monosomy 7. Subsequently, an increasing number of studies have detected missense SAMD9/SAMD9L mutations in pediatric patients with MDS, without syndromic presentations. Additionally, de Jesus and colleagues[57] detected germline frameshift SAMD9L mutations in a pediatric cohort with features that

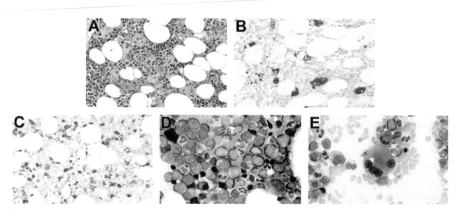

Fig. 4. Acute myeloid leukemia with germline *GATA2* mutation. Bone marrow from a 27 year old female with a history of MDS with germline GATA2 mutation with recent worsening peripheral blood counts. (*A*) The bone marrow is mildly hypocellular for age with dysplastic megakaryocytes with separated nuclear lobes and small mononuclear forms (H&E, 500×). (*B*) CD61 shows a range in size of the megakaryocytes with a subset of very small forms consistent with micromegakaryocytes (500×). (*C*) CD34 shows marked increase in CD34 positive cells, over 20%, consistent with abnormal myeloblasts identified by flow cytometry analysis of the marrow aspirate with abnormal phenotype expressing CD34, CD117, HLA-DR, CD64 (subset), cMPO, and cTDT (500×). (*D*) Bone marrow aspirate showing increased blasts with dispersed chromatin and high N:C ratio (WG stain, 1000×). (*E*) Bone marrow aspirate showing large dysplastic megakaryocyte with separated nuclear lobes (WG stain 1000×). Cytogenetics showed an abnormal karyotype with monosomy 7.

overlapped with CANDLE (autoinflammatory panniculitis resembling Chronic Atypical Neutrophilic Dermatosis with Lipodystrophy and Elevated Temperatures) syndrome. The germline mutations are gain of function resulting in negative effects on cell proliferation that favors the outgrowth of clones that have acquired revertant mutations or lost the mutant allele. The oncogenic mechanism of SAMD9/9L disorder is characterized by "adaptation by aneuploidy" that results from the nonrandom loss of chromosome 7 which contains the mutant *SAMD9/9L* gene copy.[58] Monosomy 7 increases the risk of development of MDS/AML. Importantly, somatic genetic reversion can occur in hematopoietic cells in germline *SAMD9/9L* patients resulting in restoration of normal hematopoiesis via the acquisition of truncating SAMD9/9L mutations or an independent uniparental disomy of 7q (UPD7q).[58,59] The somatic "revertant" mutations are thought to exert a loss-of-function effect thereby neutralizing the gain-of-function germline mutation. Germline *SAMD9/9L* mutations account for 8% to 17% of primary childhood MDS with a median age of 9.6 years (0.2–17.6).[58,60] The hematologic manifestations can present as cytopenias, hypocellular marrow, or MDS with −7 or del (7q). A subset of patients progress to advanced AML or CMML. Similar to pediatric *GATA2* patients, the majority of pediatric *SAM9/SAMD9L* patients present with RCC.

Myeloid Neoplasms Associated with Bone Marrow Failure Syndromes

The inherited bone marrow failure syndromes are a heterogeneous group of disorders with characteristic bone marrow dysfunction and evolving cytopenias, variable clinical presentations, and increased predisposition to MDS, AML, or isolated clonal cytogenetic alterations.

Fanconi anemia

Fanconi anemia (FA) is typically autosomal recessive with up to 22 identified *FANC* genes (*FANCB* is X-linked recessive and *FANCR/RAD21* is autosomal dominant).[61,62] Physical abnormalities are variable and may manifest as short stature, microcephaly, microphthalmia, café au-lait spots, endocrinopathies, and VACTERAL (Vertebral anomalies, anal atresia, Cardiac abnormalities, Tracheo-Esophageal fistula, renal anomalies, and radial Limb) constellation. On occasion, characteristic physical features may be subtle and their absence does not exclude FA. Bone marrow failure is frequent at a lifetime cumulative incidence of 50%, with a median age of 7 years (0–41 years).[63] Emergence of certain cytogenetic abnormalities is considered MDS defining in FA including 3q+, 7q-, –7, and complex karyotype,[64] whereas other cytogenetic abnormalities are of indeterminate potential including 1q+, 6p-, 7p-, +8, and 20q-(64). Notably, some patients present with MDS or AML without prior history of marrow failure. Patients with syndromic features are at higher risk of early onset marrow failure, whereas patients with a normal physical phenotype are more likely to develop malignancy at an older age. Squamous cell carcinoma (SCC), particularly of the skin, head and neck, and vulva, occurs at high frequencies in FA. In contrast to sporadic MDS, mutations in RUNX1 and RAS pathway genes are more common in MDS in FA patients.[65]

Shwachman-Diamond syndrome

Shwachman-Diamond syndrome (SDS) is a rare autosomal recessive, multisystem disease characterized by exocrine pancreatic insufficiency, skeletal abnormalities, impaired hematopoiesis, and increased risk of MDS and AML.[66,67] Other clinical features include skeletal, immunologic, hepatic, and cardiac disorders. Majority of affected patients are enriched in biallelic mutations in the Shwachman-Bodian-Diamond syndrome (SBDS) gene located on chromosome.[67] The SDBS protein plays a role in ribosome biogenesis and mutations impair ribosome assembly. The 20 year cumulative risk for developing severe cytopenia ranges from 9%[68] to 24.3%[69] and a 36% cumulative risk of MDS/AML at 30 years of age.[69] Bone marrow evaluation typically demonstrates hypocellular marrow with myeloid hypoplasia and mild dyspoiesis. The most common cytogenetic abnormalities are i(7q) and del (20q) that are not associated with progression to myeloid neoplasms. Xia and colleagues[70] demonstrated clonal hematopoiesis due to TP53 mutations in 48% of 27 SBS patients, which possibly serve as an early event in transformation to MDS or AML. Most SDS patients with myeloid malignancies have biallelic TP53-inactivating mutations.[66]

Telomere biology disorders including dyskeratosis congenita

Telomere biology disorders (TBDs) result from mutations in more than 14 different genes that are critical for maintenance of telomeres leading to chromosome instability and apoptosis.[71] Dyskeratosis congenita (DKC), an X-linked recessive disease, is defined by excessive telomere shortening in Xq28, where the X-linked gene *DKC1* (Dyskerin) is located. DKC is characterized by dysplastic nails, reticular skin pigmentation, and oral leukoplakia but these features may be lacking. Ninety percent of patients develop bone marrow failure by age 30 years with a high risk of hematologic and solid tumors.[72] Telomere disease is also induced by heterozygous pathogenic variants in the shelterin telomere protection complex, including *TERT, TERC, TINF2, ACD, NOP10, NHP2, WRAP53,* and *POT1,* in the DNA helicase and the telomere biology protein, *RTEL1,* a component of the telomerase holoenzyme complex, *NAF1,* and the telomere capping protein *STN1.*[71,73] Many germline TBD mutations have an autosomal dominant inheritance pattern including those affecting *TERT* (telomerase reverse transcriptase), a gene in 5p15.33, or *TERC* (telomerase RNA component), a gene in 3q26.2 with variable penetrance.[71] Flow-fluorescence in situ hybridization (FISH) for telomere length can be an informative test that typically shows teleomere length lower than the first percentile for age.[74] Clinical manifestations are variable and may present in adulthood with idiopathic pulmonary fibrosis, liver cirrhosis, early-onset gray hair, esophageal stricture and SCC of head, neck, and anogenital regions. Cytopenias, red cell macrocytosis, aplastic anemia, and evolution to MDS are observed in 30% of patients (**Fig. 5**).

Severe congenital neutropenia

Severe congenital neutropenia (SCN) are a heterogeneous group of inherited disorders of hematopoiesis characterized by impaired differentiation of neutrophilic granulocytes. Mutations in over 24 genes have been linked to congenital neutropenia including those transmitted by autosomal dominance (*ELANE, CSF3R,* and *GFI1*), autosomal recessive (*CXCR2, HAX1,* and *G6PC3*) or X-liked (*WAS*) patterns.[75] SCN caused by pathogenic variants of *ELANE* are the most frequently observed genetic alterations. Bone marrow evaluation reveals a maturation arrest at the level of promyelocytes, which generally leads to reduced neutrophil counts.[76] Eosinophilia and monocytosis may be present. A high risk of infections is frequently observed as early as in the neonatal period with an increased predisposition to MDS and AML. Recombinant granulocyte colony-stimulating factor is the treatment of choice for SCN with overall survival of 80% and reduces spontaneous risk of myeloid neoplasms.[77] Clonal hematopoiesis with acquired mutations in *CSF3R* is frequently seen in SCN patients and AML usually descends from one of these *CSF3R* mutant clones.[78] In addition, SCN patients with AML possess additional RUNX1 mutations and may require cooperating CSF3R and RUNX1 mutations for AML initiation and disease progression.[75]

Diamond-Blackfan anemia

Diamond-Blackfan anemia (DBA) is a rare inherited bone marrow failure disease, resulting from loss-of-function mutations/deletions in 1 of 23 genes encoding either a small or a large subunit-associated ribosomal protein (eg, *RPS19, RPS17, RPS24, RPL35 A, RPL5, RPL11, RPS7, RPS26 RPS10*).[79] DBA may be inherited in autosomal dominant in 45% of cases and the remainder of the mutations are sporadic and appear to represent new dominant cases. DBA is characterized by severe macrocytic anemia in infancy, reticulocytopenia, and elevated erythrocyte adenosine deaminase.[80] Congenital anomalies are highly variable and include short stature, webbed neck, thumb abnormalities, genitourinary, and hearing defects. Cumulative incidence of MDS/AML and solid tumors reaches 20% at the age of 46 years.[80] The bone marrow is normocellular or mildly hypocellular with marked erythroid hypoplasia. Immature erythroid precursors may be prominent with maturation arrest and diminished mature forms. Dyserythropoiesis is not uncommon and other lineages are unaffected. Spontaneous remission may be observed in 25% of DBA patients. HSCT may be reserved for patients unresponsive to corticosteroids or those who develop myeloid neoplasms.[80]

Juvenile myelomonocytic leukemia

Juvenile myelomonocytic leukemia (JMML), a myeloproliferative/myelodysplastic disorder, is associated with genetic alterations in components of the *RAS/MAPK* signal transduction pathway including *NRAS, KRAS, PTPN11, NF1, CBL* or rarely *RRAS*. Germline mutations (inherited or occurring *de novo*) predisposing to JMML occurs in approximately 25% of cases.[81] The WHO 2016 diagnostic criteria for JMML include peripheral blood monocyte count of greater than or equal to 1×10^9/L, splenomegaly,

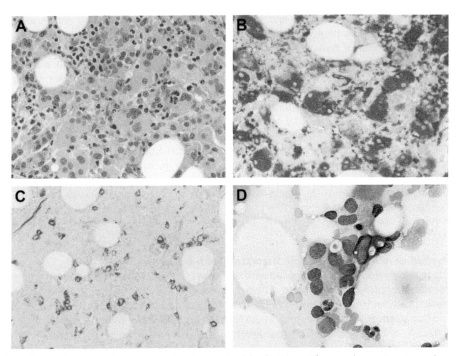

Fig. 5. Myelodysplastic syndrome/acute myeloid leukemia with germline *TERT* mutation. Marrow from a male in his 50s with a history of pancytopenia, pulmonary fibrosis, early graying of the hair, and germline mutation in *TERT*. (*A*) Hypercellular marrow with increased dysplastic megakaryocytes and increased immature precursors (H&E, 500×). (*B*). CD61 immunostain highlighting increased dysplastic megakaryocytes (500×). (*C*) CD34 showing increased positive cells (15% overall) consistent with abnormal myeloblasts expressing CD7 confirmed by flow cytometry analysis (500×). (*D*) Aspirate smear showing dysplastic megakaryocytes and blasts (WG stain, 1000×).

blast count less than 20%, and absence of *BCR/ABL1* translocation.[82] The International Consensus Classification (ICC) of 2022 now requires a RAS pathway mutation for diagnosis of JMML, and notes that a subset of patients may not have splenomegaly or monocytosis in the early stages of disease[8,83,84] The updated WHO 5th edition classification does not require a RAS pathway mutation for diagnosis.[10,85] JMML cases in general develop thrombocytopenia with exception of NF1-associated JMML.[9,86] Bone marrow is hypercellular with myeloid hyperplasia and less prominent monocytosis in comparison to the peripheral blood and decreased number of megakaryocytes. Monosomy of chromosome 7 is the most common karyotype aberration in JMML and is most frequent in *KRAS* mutated JMML. The hallmark of JMML is the constitutional activation of *RAS* signaling pathway. Three subtypes are recognized.[86] The *PTPN11, NRAS,* and *KRAS* mutated JMML that are defined by heterozygous somatic gain-of-function mutations without constitutional syndromes. The remaining 2 subtypes including JMML associated with neurofibromatosis and JMML with *CBL* syndrome are defined by germline Ras disease and acquired biallelic inactivation of the respective genes in hematopoietic cells. Children with neoplasms resembling JMML without *RAS*-pathway mutations are classified as JMML-like in the ICC.

Neurofibromatosis type I (NF1), an autosomal dominant disorder, is caused by mutations in neurofibromin 1 gene (*NF1*), a negative regulator of *RAS*.[81] Clinical symptoms increase over time and multiple café au lait spots, axillary and inguinal freckling, cutaneous neurofibromas, iris Lisch nodules, and choroidal freckling are frequent. The risk of benign and malignant tumors is high in these individuals with 200 to 500 times more likely to develop JMML. Patients with NF1 can develop JMML after acquiring loss of heterozygosity (LOH) via uniparental isodisomy with loss of the wild-type NF1 allele and duplication of the mutant allele.[87] LOH may occur less frequently through compound-heterozygous NF1-inactivating mutations or somatic interstitial deletions. Fatal outcomes are observed in this subtype without allogeneic HSCT.[86]

Juvenile myelomonocytic leukemia associated with Noonan-syndrome-like disorder (CBL syndrome), and Noonan syndrome (NS) is a genetic disease with characteristic features of facial dysmorphism, growth delay, and heart disease.[31] NS patients develop JMML, typically at young age that may regress spontaneously over time. Germline mutations affecting *PTPN11, RIT1, RRAS, and SOS1* have been described in patients with Noonan syndrome, some of which also may develop features of JMML.[88,89]

Myeloid or lymphoid neoplasms associated with Down syndrome

The myeloid neoplasms associated with germline trisomy 21 (Down syndrome) are the transient abnormal myelopoiesis (TAM) and AML.[90] Most TAM cases spontaneously resolve without treatment and around 10% acquire additional cooperating mutations and transform to AML. Mutations in *GATA1*, which cooperate with the underlying trisomy 21, are associated with the development of TAM in Down syndrome.[91] The development of AML is associated with additional acquired mutation(s), often in genes encoding cohesins, or those involved in the JAK-STAT signaling pathway.[92] Majority of the AML cases are acute megakaryoblastic leukemia, which accounts for 50% of cases. AML is often preceded by a prolonged MDS-like phase characterized by thrombocytopenia, subsequent anemia, and bone marrow dysplasia. Patients with Down syndrome also have an increased risk of B-ALL.[93]

SUMMARY

Recognition of hematologic neoplasms with germline predisposition is important for both clinicians and pathologists. The field is actively evolving due to the widespread availability of next generation sequencing methods for myeloid neoplasms revealing that germline predisposition is more common than previously thought. Additional novel genetic mutations continue to be discovered and will likely be incorporated into future diagnostic classifications as compelling evidence emerges. Additional genes that may be added include *ERCC6L2, MECOM, BLM, LIG4, XPC, DNMT3A, TET2,* and *CSF3R* and genes involved in constitutional mismatch repair deficiency *(MLH1, MSH2, MSH6, EPCAM, PNS2), BLM* was recently added to the updated WHO 5th edition classification.

Some of the genes predisposing to myeloid malignancy show variable penetrance and expressivity. Heterozygous germline carriers may present with cytopenias with varying degrees of dyspoiesis at the baseline bone marrow evaluation that may be related to the genetic disease pathology and not indicative of MDS. In patients with germline mutations in genes associated with inherited thrombocytopenia (RUNX1, ANKRD26, and ETV6), dysmegakaryopoiesis is very common and in the setting of isolated thrombocytopenia should not be considered as criteria for MDS. Importantly, before a diagnosis of MDS is rendered it is helpful to have additional findings supporting a diagnosis of MDS or myeloid malignancy including overt multilineage dysplasia, ring sideroblasts, increased blasts, cytogenetic abnormalities, or acquired somatic mutations supporting a diagnosis of myeloid malignancy. HSCT is often the treatment of choice and if a related donor is considered, the donor should be tested for the patient's germline mutation regardless of the health of the donor, in order to avoid donor derived MDS/AML post-transplant. Certain predisposition syndromes such as JMML with CBL syndrome undergo spontaneous remission and do not require transplant.

The key to diagnosis of these familial syndromes is the detection of the germline mutation. Many cases are initially suspected when mutations are identified with high VAFs in the range of 30% to 60%, during sequencing analysis of hematologic malignancies in bone marrow or blood on NGS panels. Confirmation of a suspected germline mutation ideally requires testing on a germline tissue source, the gold standard for which is cultured fibroblasts from a skin biopsy. Buccal swabs are often contaminated with hematopoietic cells. Nail clippings can be contaminated by monocytes. Hair follicles may not result in sufficient DNA. A positive germline mutation can be inferred if the same mutation is detected in a first-degree relative, or if the mutation persists at a high VAF at serial time points after chemotherapy. Certain mutations in non-coding regions may be missed by whole exome sequencing or targeted NGS panels and may benefit from additional testing for non-coding or pathogenic synonymous mutations, or large deletions/insertions. In general, the presence of MDS or AML in children and adolescents should prompt an evaluation for germline mutations to determine early risk assessment and development of effective therapies.

CLINICS CARE POINTS

- Germline mutations may be detected on targeted myeloid mutation panels designed for somatic mutations if the region of the mutation is covered on the panel.
- In general, germline mutations have VAFs close to 50% but can range from 30% to 60%.
- If somatic genetic rescue occurs in hematopoietic cells, the VAF of the germline mutation may be very low; therefore, a VAF less than 30% does not rule out a germline mutation.
- A persistently high VAF in a gene, detected in a patient's marrow/blood pre- and post-chemotherapy at serial timepoints, suggests possible germline mutation.
- In the blood/marrow of a patient with a hematologic malignancy, both somatic and germline mutations can have high VAFs, making it hard to distinguish somatic from germline mutations.
- A suspected germline mutation detected in blood/marrow from a patient with a hematologic malignancy should be confirmed on a germline tissue source such as cultured fibroblasts from a skin biopsy (gold standard). Buccal swabs may be contaminated with blood cells. Nail clippings may contain monocytes. Hair follicles may not yield enough DNA.
- If the same mutation is detected in the patient and another family member, this supports a germline mutation.
- Biallelic mutations detected in a hematologic malignancy in genes associated with germline predisposition (eg, RUNX1, CEBPA, or DDX41) raises the possibility of a germline mutation and a second somatic mutation.

CONFLICT OF INTEREST STATEMENT

The authors have nothing to disclose.

ACKNOWLEDGMENTS

This work was in part funded by the National Institutes of Health, Intramural Research Program, of the NIH Clinical Center.

REFERENCES

1. Gao J, Chen Y, Sukhanova M. Molecular pathogenesis in myeloid neoplasms with germline predisposition. Life 2021;12(1):46.
2. Galera P, Hsu AP, Wang W, et al. Donor-derived MDS/AML in families with germline GATA2 mutation. Blood 2018;132(18):1994–8.
3. Kobayashi S, Kobayashi A, Osawa Y, et al. Donor cell leukemia arising from pre-leukemic clones with a novel germline DDX41 mutation after allogenic hematopoietic stem cell transplantation. Leukemia 2017;31(4):1020–2.
4. Xiao H, Shi J, Luo Y, et al. First report of multiple CEBPA mutations contributing to donor origin of leukemia relapse after allogeneic hematopoietic stem cell transplantation. Blood 2011;117(19):5257–60.
5. Owen CJ, Toze CL, Koochin A, et al. Five new pedigrees with inherited RUNX1 mutations causing familial platelet disorder with propensity to myeloid malignancy. Blood 2008;112(12):4639–45.
6. Acuna-Hidalgo R, Veltman JA, Hoischen A. New insights into the generation and role of de novo mutations in health and disease. Genome Biol 2016;17(1):241.
7. Duncavage EJ, Bagg A, Hasserjian RP, et al. Genomic profiling for clinical decision making in myeloid neoplasms and acute leukemia. Blood 2022;140(21):2228–47.
8. Arber DA, Orazi A, Hasserjian R, et al. The 2016 revision to the World Health Organization classification of myeloid neoplasms and acute leukemia. Blood 2016;127(20):2391–405.
9. Arber DA, Orazi A, Hasserjian RP, et al. International Consensus classification of myeloid neoplasms and acute leukemias: integrating morphologic, clinical, and genomic data. Blood 2022;140(11):1200–28.
10. Khoury JD, Solary E, Abla O, et al. The 5th edition of the world health organization classification of haematolymphoid Tumours: myeloid and histiocytic/dendritic neoplasms. Leukemia 2022;36(7):1703–19.
11. Zhang P, Iwasaki-Arai J, Iwasaki H, et al. Enhancement of hematopoietic stem cell repopulating capacity and self-renewal in the absence of the transcription factor C/EBP alpha. Immunity 2004;21(6):853–63.
12. Pabst T, Mueller BU, Zhang P, et al. Dominant-negative mutations of CEBPA, encoding CCAAT/enhancer binding protein-alpha (C/EBPalpha), in acute myeloid leukemia. Nat Genet 2001;27(3):263–70.
13. Zhang Y, Wang F, Chen X, et al. Companion gene mutations and their clinical significance in AML with double mutant CEBPA. Cancer Gene Ther 2020;27(7–8):599–606.
14. Tawana K, Wang J, Renneville A, et al. Disease evolution and outcomes in familial AML with germline CEBPA mutations. Blood 2015;126(10):1214–23.
15. Pabst T, Eyholzer M, Haefliger S, et al. Somatic CEBPA mutations are a frequent second event in families with germline CEBPA mutations and familial acute myeloid leukemia. J Clin Oncol 2008;26(31):5088–93.
16. Andreou AZ. DDX41: a multifunctional DEAD-box protein involved in pre-mRNA splicing and innate immunity. Biol Chem 2021;402(5):645–51.
17. Shinriki S, Matsui H. Unique role of DDX41, a DEAD-box type RNA helicase, in hematopoiesis and leukemogenesis. Frontiers in oncology 2022;12:992340.

18. Li P, Brown S, Williams M, et al. The genetic landscape of germline DDX41 variants predisposing to myeloid neoplasms. Blood 2022;140(7):716–55.
19. Lewinsohn M, Brown AL, Weinel LM, et al. Novel germ line DDX41 mutations define families with a lower age of MDS/AML onset and lymphoid malignancies. Blood 2016;127(8):1017–23.
20. Petitjean A, Achatz MI, Borresen-Dale AL, et al. TP53 mutations in human cancers: functional selection and impact on cancer prognosis and outcomes. Oncogene 2007;26(15):2157–65.
21. Li FP, Fraumeni JF Jr, Mulvihill JJ, et al. A cancer family syndrome in twenty-four kindreds. Cancer Res 1988;48(18):5358–62.
22. Bougeard G, Renaux-Petel M, Flaman JM, et al. Revisiting Li-fraumeni syndrome from TP53 mutation carriers. J Clin Oncol 2015;33(21):2345–52.
23. Holmfeldt L, Wei L, Diaz-Flores E, et al. The genomic landscape of hypodiploid acute lymphoblastic leukemia. Nat Genet 2013;45(3):242–52.
24. Link DC, Schuettpelz LG, Shen D, et al. Identification of a novel TP53 cancer susceptibility mutation through whole-genome sequencing of a patient with therapy-related AML. JAMA 2011;305(15):1568–76.
25. Harrison CJ, Moorman AV, Broadfield ZJ, et al. Three distinct subgroups of hypodiploidy in acute lymphoblastic leukaemia. Br J Haematol 2004;125(5):552–9.
26. Song WJ, Sullivan MG, Legare RD, et al. Haploinsufficiency of CBFA2 causes familial thrombocytopenia with propensity to develop acute myelogenous leukaemia. Nat Genet 1999;23(2):166–75.
27. Brown AL, Arts P, Carmichael CL, et al. RUNX1-mutated families show phenotype heterogeneity and a somatic mutation profile unique to germline predisposed AML. Blood advances 2020;4(6):1131–44.
28. Schlegelberger B, Heller PG. RUNX1 deficiency (familial platelet disorder with predisposition to myeloid leukemia, FPDMM). Semin Hematol 2017;54(2):75–80.
29. Bluteau D, Glembotsky AC, Raimbault A, et al. Dysmegakaryopoiesis of FPD/AML pedigrees with constitutional RUNX1 mutations is linked to myosin II deregulated expression. Blood 2012;120(13):2708–18.
30. Kanagal-Shamanna R, Loghavi S, DiNardo CD, et al. Bone marrow pathologic abnormalities in familial platelet disorder with propensity for myeloid malignancy and germline RUNX1 mutation. Haematologica 2017;102(10):1661–70.
31. Klco JM, Mulligan CG. Advances in germline predisposition to acute leukaemias and myeloid neoplasms. Nat Rev Cancer 2021;21(2):122–37.
32. Pippucci T, Savoia A, Perrotta S, et al. Mutations in the 5' UTR of ANKRD26, the ankirin repeat domain 26 gene, cause an autosomal-dominant form of inherited thrombocytopenia, THC2. Am J Hum Genet 2011;88(1):115–20.
33. Bluteau D, Balduini A, Balayn N, et al. Thrombocytopenia-associated mutations in the ANKRD26 regulatory region induce MAPK hyperactivation. J Clin Invest 2014; 124(2):580–91.
34. Noris P, Perrotta S, Seri M, et al. Mutations in ANKRD26 are responsible for a frequent form of inherited thrombocytopenia: analysis of 78 patients from 21 families. Blood 2011;117(24):6673–80.
35. Zaninetti C, Santini V, Tiniakou M, et al. Inherited thrombocytopenia caused by ANKRD26 mutations misdiagnosed and treated as myelodysplastic syndrome: report on two cases. J Thromb Haemost 2017;15(12):2388–92.
36. Noris P, Favier R, Alessi MC, et al. ANKRD26-related thrombocytopenia and myeloid malignancies. Blood 2013;122(11):1987–9.

37. Golub TR, Barker GF, Lovett M, et al. Fusion of PDGF receptor beta to a novel ets-like gene, tel, in chronic myelomonocytic leukemia with t(5;12) chromosomal translocation. Cell 1994;77(2):307–16.
38. Zhang MY, Churpek JE, Keel SB, et al. Germline ETV6 mutations in familial thrombocytopenia and hematologic malignancy. Nat Genet 2015;47(2):180–5.
39. Noetzli L, Lo RW, Lee-Sherick AB, et al. Germline mutations in ETV6 are associated with thrombocytopenia, red cell macrocytosis and predisposition to lymphoblastic leukemia. Nat Genet 2015;47(5):535–8.
40. Topka S, Vijai J, Walsh MF, et al. Germline ETV6 mutations confer susceptibility to acute lymphoblastic leukemia and thrombocytopenia. PLoS Genet 2015;11(6): e1005262.
41. Feurstein S, Godley LA. Germline ETV6 mutations and predisposition to hematological malignancies. Int J Hematol 2017;106(2):189–95.
42. Hsu AP, Sampaio EP, Khan J, et al. Mutations in GATA2 are associated with the autosomal dominant and sporadic monocytopenia and mycobacterial infection (MonoMAC) syndrome. Blood 2011;118(10):2653–5.
43. Dickinson RE, Griffin H, Bigley V, et al. Exome sequencing identifies GATA-2 mutation as the cause of dendritic cell, monocyte, B and NK lymphoid deficiency. Blood 2011;118(10):2656–8.
44. Hahn CN, Chong CE, Carmichael CL, et al. Heritable GATA2 mutations associated with familial myelodysplastic syndrome and acute myeloid leukemia. Nat Genet 2011;43(10):1012–7.
45. Ostergaard P, Simpson MA, Connell FC, et al. Mutations in GATA2 cause primary lymphedema associated with a predisposition to acute myeloid leukemia (Emberger syndrome). Nat Genet 2011;43(10):929–31.
46. Spinner MA, Sanchez LA, Hsu AP, et al. GATA2 deficiency: a protean disorder of hematopoiesis, lymphatics, and immunity. Blood 2014;123(6):809–21.
47. Vicente C, Conchillo A, García-Sánchez MA, et al. The role of the GATA2 transcription factor in normal and malignant hematopoiesis. Crit Rev Oncol Hematol 2012;82(1):1–17.
48. Rodrigues NP, Janzen V, Forkert R, et al. Haploinsufficiency of GATA-2 perturbs adult hematopoietic stem-cell homeostasis. Blood 2005;106(2):477–84.
49. Calvo KR, Hickstein DD. The spectrum of GATA2 deficiency syndrome. Blood 2023;141(13):1524–32.
50. Ganapathi KA, Townsley DM, Hsu AP, et al. GATA2 deficiency-associated bone marrow disorder differs from idiopathic aplastic anemia. Blood 2015;125(1): 56–70.
51. Sahoo SS, Kozyra EJ, Wlodarski MW. Germline predisposition in myeloid neoplasms: unique genetic and clinical features of GATA2 deficiency and SAMD9/ SAMD9L syndromes. Best Pract Res Clin Haematol 2020;33(3):101197.
52. Wlodarski MW, Hirabayashi S, Pastor V, et al. Prevalence, clinical characteristics, and prognosis of GATA2-related myelodysplastic syndromes in children and adolescents. Blood 2016;127(11):1387–97, quiz 518.
53. McReynolds LJ, Calvo KR, Holland SM. Germline GATA2 mutation and bone marrow failure. Hematol Oncol Clin N Am 2018;32(4):713–28.
54. Hsu AP, Johnson KD, Falcone EL, et al. GATA2 haploinsufficiency caused by mutations in a conserved intronic element leads to MonoMAC syndrome. Blood 2013;121(19):3830–7.
55. Narumi S, Amano N, Ishii T, et al. SAMD9 mutations cause a novel multisystem disorder, MIRAGE syndrome, and are associated with loss of chromosome 7. Nat Genet 2016;48(7):792–7.

56. Chen DH, Below JE, Shimamura A, et al. Ataxia-pancytopenia syndrome is caused by missense mutations in SAMD9L. Am J Hum Genet 2016;98(6):1146–58.

57. de Jesus AA, Hou Y, Brooks S, et al. Distinct interferon signatures and cytokine patterns define additional systemic autoinflammatory diseases. The Journal of clinical investigation 2020;130(4):1669–82.

58. Wong JC, Bryant V, Lamprecht T, et al. Germline SAMD9 and SAMD9L mutations are associated with extensive genetic evolution and diverse hematologic outcomes. JCI insight 2018;3(14):e121086.

59. Victor BP, Sushree SS, Jessica B, et al. Constitutional SAMD9L mutations cause familial myelodysplastic syndrome and transient monosomy 7. Haematologica 2018;103(3):427–37.

60. Sahoo SS, Pastor Loyola V, Panda PK, et al. SAMD9 and SAMD9L germline disorders in patients enrolled in studies of the European working group of MDS in childhood (EWOG-MDS): prevalence, outcome, phenotype and functional characterisation. Blood 2018;132(Supplement 1):643.

61. Avagyan S, Shimamura A. Lessons from pediatric MDS: approaches to germline predisposition to hematologic malignancies. Frontiers in oncology 2022;12:813149.

62. Groarke EM, Young NS, Calvo KR. Distinguishing constitutional from acquired bone marrow failure in the hematology clinic. Best Pract Res Clin Haematol 2021;34(2):101275.

63. Alter BP. Fanconi anemia and the development of leukemia. Best Pract Res Clin Haematol 2014;27(3–4):214–21.

64. Behrens YL, Gohring G, Bawadi R, et al. A novel classification of hematologic conditions in patients with Fanconi anemia. Haematologica 2021;106(11):3000–3.

65. Chao MM, Thomay K, Goehring G, et al. Mutational spectrum of fanconi anemia associated myeloid neoplasms. Klin Pädiatr 2017;229(6):329–34.

66. Reilly CR, Shimamura A. Predisposition to myeloid malignancies in Shwachman-Diamond syndrome: biological insights and clinical advances. Blood 2023;141(13):1513–23.

67. Furutani E, Liu S, Galvin A, et al. Hematologic complications with age in Shwachman-Diamond syndrome. Blood Adv 2022;6(1):297–306.

68. Cesaro S, Pegoraro A, Sainati L, et al. A prospective study of hematologic complications and long-term survival of Italian patients affected by shwachman-diamond syndrome. J Pediatr 2020;219:196–201.e1.

69. Donadieu J, Fenneteau O, Beaupain B, et al. Classification of and risk factors for hematologic complications in a French national cohort of 102 patients with Shwachman-Diamond syndrome. Haematologica 2012;97(9):1312–9.

70. Xia J, Miller CA, Baty J, et al. Somatic mutations and clonal hematopoiesis in congenital neutropenia. Blood 2018;131(4):408–16.

71. Grill S, Nandakumar J. Molecular mechanisms of telomere biology disorders. J Biol Chem 2021;296:100064.

72. Calado RT, Young NS. Telomere diseases. N Engl J Med 2009;361(24):2353–65.

73. Niewisch MR, Savage SA. An update on the biology and management of dyskeratosis congenita and related telomere biology disorders. Expert Rev Hematol 2019;12(12):1037–52.

74. Armanios M, Blackburn EH. The telomere syndromes. Nat Rev Genet 2012;13(10):693–704.

75. Skokowa J, Dale DC, Touw IP, et al. Severe congenital neutropenias. Nat Rev Dis Prim 2017;3:17032.

Obiorah et al

76. Welte K, Zeidler C, Dale DC. Severe congenital neutropenia. Semin Hematol 2006;43(3):189–95.
77. Rosenberg PS, Zeidler C, Bolyard AA, et al. Stable long-term risk of leukaemia in patients with severe congenital neutropenia maintained on G-CSF therapy. Br J Haematol 2010;150(2):196–9.
78. Touw IP. Game of clones: the genomic evolution of severe congenital neutropenia. Hematology Am Soc Hematol Educ Program 2015;2015:1–7.
79. Ulirsch JC, Verboon JM, Kazerounian S, et al. The genetic landscape of diamond-blackfan anemia. Am J Hum Genet 2018;103(6):930–47.
80. Vlachos A, Muir E. How I treat Diamond-Blackfan anemia. Blood 2010;116(19):3715–23.
81. Wintering A, Dvorak CC, Stieglitz E, et al. Juvenile myelomonocytic leukemia in the molecular era: a clinician's guide to diagnosis, risk stratification, and treatment. Blood advances 2021;5(22):4783–93.
82. Swerdlow SH, Campo E, Harris NL, et al. WHO classification of Tumours of the haematopoietic and lymphoid tissues. Lyon Cedex, France: International Agency for Research on Cancer; 2017.
83. Rudelius M, Weinberg OK, Niemeyer CM, et al. The International Consensus Classification (ICC) of hematologic neoplasms with germline predisposition, pediatric myelodysplastic syndrome, and juvenile myelomonocytic leukemia. Virchows Arch 2023;482(1):113–30.
84. Niemeyer CM, Rudelius M, Shimamura A, et al. Classification of rare pediatric myeloid neoplasia-Quo vadis? Leukemia 2022;36(12):2947–8.
85. Elghetany MT, Cave H, De Vito R, et al. Juvenile myelomonocytic leukemia; moving forward. Leukemia 2023;37(3):720–2.
86. Niemeyer CM, Flotho C. Juvenile myelomonocytic leukemia: who's the driver at the wheel? Blood 2019;133(10):1060–70.
87. Steinemann D, Arning L, Praulich I, et al. Mitotic recombination and compound-heterozygous mutations are predominant NF1-inactivating mechanisms in children with juvenile myelomonocytic leukemia and neurofibromatosis type 1. Haematologica 2010;95(2):320–3.
88. Niemeyer CM. JMML genomics and decisions. Hematology Am Soc Hematol Educ Program 2018;2018(1):307–12.
89. O'Halloran K, Ritchey AK, Djokic M, et al. Transient juvenile myelomonocytic leukemia in the setting of PTPN11 mutation and Noonan syndrome with secondary development of monosomy 7. Pediatr Blood Cancer 2017;64(7):1–4.
90. Hitzler JK, Zipursky A. Origins of leukaemia in children with Down syndrome. Nat Rev Cancer 2005;5(1):11–20.
91. Labuhn M, Perkins K, Matzk S, et al. Mechanisms of progression of myeloid pre-leukemia to transformed myeloid leukemia in children with Down syndrome. Cancer Cell 2019;36(2):123–138 e10.
92. Kratz CP, Izraeli S. Down syndrome, RASopathies, and other rare syndromes. Semin Hematol 2017;54(2):123–8.
93. Izraeli S. The acute lymphoblastic leukemia of Down Syndrome - genetics and pathogenesis. Eur J Med Genet 2016;59(3):158–61.

Childhood Myelodysplastic Syndrome

Karen M. Chisholm, MD, PhD[a,b],*, Sandra D. Bohling, MD[a,b]

KEYWORDS

- Childhood myelodysplastic syndrome (MDS)
- Inherited bone marrow failure syndrome • Germline predisposition • MDS
- Myelodysplastic syndrome • Refractory cytopenia of childhood • Pediatric MDS

KEY POINTS

- Myelodysplastic syndrome (MDS) is very rare in childhood.
- Current terminology includes refractory cytopenia of childhood (RCC)/MDS with low blasts (cMDS-LB) for cases with < 2% peripheral blood and < 5% bone marrow blasts and MDS-excess blasts/MDS-increased blasts for cases with ≥2% peripheral blood or ≥5% bone marrow blasts.
- The most common diagnosis in children is RCC/cMDS-LB, of which ~80% have hypocellular bone marrows.
- Molecular analysis has revealed underlying germline predisposing mutations in 24% to 31% of cases and different somatic signatures (enrichment in RAS pathway mutations) when compared with adult MDS.
- Therapeutic strategies are dependent on the clinical scenario and include watch-and-wait, immunosuppressive therapy, and hematopoietic stem cell transplant (HSCT). HSCT is the only curative treatment.

INTRODUCTION/CLASSIFICATION

Myelodysplastic syndrome (MDS) is an acquired clonal hematopoietic stem cell disorder characterized by ineffective hematopoiesis, as evidenced by cytopenias, morphologic dysplasia, and risk for progression to acute myeloid leukemia. Childhood MDS (cMDS) can either be primary ("de novo") or secondary, with secondary MDS being associated with antecedent or predisposing conditions such as certain genetic mutations, inherited bone marrow failure syndromes (IBMFSs), prior chemotherapy/radiation therapy (therapy-related MDS), or acquired severe aplastic anemia. Compared with adults, MDS in childhood and adolescents (defined as <18 years of age) is far

ᵃ Hematopathology, Department of Laboratories, Seattle Children's Hospital, 4800 Sand Point Way Northeast, FB.4.510, Seattle, WA 98105, USA; ᵇ Department of Laboratory Medicine and Pathology, University of Washington Medical Center, 4800 Sand Point Way Northeast, FB.4.510, Seattle, WA 98105, USA
* Corresponding author.
E-mail address: karen.chisholm@seattlechildrens.org

Clin Lab Med 43 (2023) 639–655
https://doi.org/10.1016/j.cll.2023.06.005
0272-2712/23/© 2023 Elsevier Inc. All rights reserved.
labmed.theclinics.com

less common, uses different terminology, and has been shown to be biologically distinct.[1,2] Two hematopathology classification systems are currently used for the categorization of MDS: the recently released International Consensus Classification (ICC)[3,4] and the 5th edition of the World Health Organization (WHO)[5]; both will be referenced below.

Some of the unique terminology currently used in cMDS was introduced in 2003 when Hasle and colleagues[6] proposed the term "refractory cytopenia" for pediatric cases of MDS without elevated blast counts and reserved a diagnosis of MDS for patients with increased blasts. The rationale for omitting "MDS" from the terminology for low-grade cases stems from the knowledge that dysplasia is often seen in benign pediatric settings such as infections, metabolic diseases, and nutritional deficiencies. This classification was incorporated into the 2008 WHO hematopoietic classification with the provisional entity "refractory cytopenia of childhood" (RCC).[7] RCC remained a provisional entity in the 2016 WHO hematopoietic neoplasm classification[8] and included cases with multilineage dysplasia.[7]

The 5th edition of the WHO replaces RCC with "childhood MDS with low blasts" (cMDS-LB).[5] This category encompasses two myelodysplastic neoplasm subtypes characterized by < 5% blasts in the bone marrow and < 2% in the peripheral blood: (1) cMDS-LB, hypocellular and (2) cMDS-LB, not otherwise specified (NOS).[5] For cases with $\geq$5% blasts in the bone marrow and/or $\geq$2% blasts in the peripheral blood, the WHO created the "childhood MDS with increased blasts" (cMDS-IB) category.[5] In contrast, the ICC retained the terminology of RCC for cases meeting defined morphologic criteria including < 2% blasts in the peripheral blood and < 5% blasts in the bone marrow (**Tables 1** and **2**).[3,4] Dysplastic features are defined in RCC as either: (1) dysplasia in > 1 cell lineage or (2) dysplasia in > 10% of cells in one lineage. Cases that do not have the classic morphology of RCC and do not have increased blasts are classified as MDS-NOS.[4] This latter category also encompasses cases without cytopenias and/or dysplasia but harboring MDS-defining cytogenetic abnormalities such as monosomy 7. The ICC classifies pediatric MDS with peripheral blood blasts between 2% and 19% and/or bone marrow blasts between 5% and 19% as MDS with excess blasts (MDS-EB).[4] Of note, many cases of acute myeloid leukemia (AML) with recurrent genetic abnormalities no longer require a 20% blast count; therefore, exclusion of such rearrangements and genetic mutations is required for cMDS-IB and MDS-EB.[4,5]

In the era of next-generation sequencing (NGS), many gene mutations have been identified which predispose to MDS; these mutations are far more common in cMDS compared with adult MDS.[2,9,10] Both the WHO and ICC now include separate classifications for MDS with germline mutations: myeloid neoplasms with germline predisposition (WHO)[5] or hematologic neoplasms with germline predisposition (ICC).[3,4]

Therapy-related MDS in children encompasses a minority of MDS cases (7%–8%).[11] Similar to adults, these cases occur after receiving cytotoxic chemotherapy (such as alkylating agents and topoisomerase II inhibitors) and/or radiation. Children with a history of treatment for solid tumors (such as neuroblastoma or Ewing sarcoma) have an incidence of therapy-related MDS or AML of up to 11%,[12,13] whereas pediatric patients treated for acute lymphoblastic leukemia have a lower incidence (<3%).[14,15] In the WHO 5th edition,[5] therapy-related MDS is termed myeloid neoplasm post cytotoxic therapy, whereas the ICC[3] adds a qualifier of "therapy-related" after the MDS diagnosis.

EPIDEMIOLOGY

MDS is quite uncommon in children, accounting for < 5% of all hematologic malignancies diagnosed in this age group.[6,16,17] The annual incidence of MDS in children

Table 1
World Health Organization 5th edition and International Consensus Classification definitions of childhood myelodysplastic syndrome

WHO 5th Edition Classification		cMDS-LB	cMDS-IB
ICC classification	**RCC**	**MDS, NOS**	**MDS-EB**
Cytopenias	1–3 lineages	0–3 lineages	0–3 lineages
Dysplasia Morphology	≥2 lineages OR ≥1 lineage, involving at least 10% of cells Typical histologic features of RCC[a]	0–3 lineages Do not have typical histology of RCC	0–3 lineage, involving at least 10% of cells
Peripheral blood blasts	<2%	<2%	2%–19%
Bone marrow blasts	<5%	<5%	5%–19%
Cytogenetics	Any, but excluding AML-defining cytogenetics	Any, but excluding AML-defining cytogenetics; includes MDS-defining abnormalities when there are no cytopenias or dysplasia	Any, but excluding AML-defining cytogenetics or molecular alterations
Other	No fibrosis No prior cytotoxic chemotherapy or radiation therapy		

Abbreviations: AML, acute myeloid leukemia; cMDS, childhood myelodysplastic syndrome; EB, excess blasts; IB, increased blasts; ICC, International Consensus Classification; LB, low blasts; MDS, myelodysplastic syndrome; NOS, not otherwise specified; RCC, refractory cytopenia of childhood; WHO, World Health Organization.
   [a] Typical features of RCC include hypocellular marrow (~80% of cases), patchy erythroid islands (composed of >20 cells) showing abnormal paratrabecular localization and increased mitotic activity, and megakaryocytic hypoplasia with micromegakaryocytes.
   Adapted from references[3–5]

aged 1 to 14 years has been calculated at 1 to 2 cases per million children.[6,11,16,17] cMDS without excess blasts (RCC, MDS, NOS, and cMDS-LB) is the most common MDS in childhood, accounting for > 50% of cases.[11,18] Although the median age at diagnosis is approximately 7 to 8 years, MDS can present in children of any age.[19–23] The male-to-female ratio is approximately equal.[17,19–24]

PRESENTATION AND LABORATORY FINDINGS

cMDS is usually characterized by persistent cytopenias. In RCC/cMDS-LB, thrombocytopenia (<150 × 10^9/L) is the most common, present in ~75%, followed by anemia (<10 g/dL) in ~50%, neutropenia (<1.0 × 10^9/L) in ~50%, and severe neutropenia (0.5 × 10^9/L) in ~25% of those affected.[6,21] The anemia is frequently macrocytic with an elevated mean corpuscular volume (MCV) in 75% to 90% of cases.[6,21] Hemoglobin F can also be elevated.[21] Presenting symptoms typically reflect the cytopenias and commonly include malaise, increased bleeding, fever, and infections; however, up to 20% of patients may be asymptomatic.[21] Lymphadenopathy is uncommon and,

Table 2
Hypocellular refractory cytopenia of childhood/childhood myelodysplastic neoplasms-low blasts versus severe aplastic anemia

	Hypocellular RCC/cMDS-LB	Severe Aplastic Anemia
Cytopenias	≥1 lineage	≥2 lineages: ANC <500/μL, Platelets <20 K/μL, and/or reticulocyte count <20 K/μL or <1% corrected for hematocrit
Peripheral blood blasts	<2%	<2%
Marrow cellularity	Hypocellular, often 5%–10% of cellularity for age	<25%; often <5%
Bone marrow blasts	<5%	<5%
Dysplasia	≥2 lineages OR ≥1 lineage, involving at least 10% of cells	Lack of dysplastic features
Erythropoiesis	Aspirate smears: • Dysplastic features include nuclear budding and multinucleation • Megaloblastoid changes Core biopsy: • Patchy distribution with large islands of ≥20 cells • Left-shifted maturation • Increased mitotic figures • Abnormal localization	Aspirate smears: • Markedly decreased in number • Lack of dysplastic features • Lack of megaloblastoid changes Core biopsy: • Markedly decreased in number • If islands present, <10 cells • Full-spectrum maturation
Myelopoiesis	Aspirate smears: • Markedly decreased in number • Left-shifted maturation • Dysplastic features include pseudo-Pelger-Huët nuclei, hypogranular cytoplasm, and nuclear-to-cytoplasmic dyssynchrony Core biopsy: • Markedly decreased in number • Left-shifted maturation • Intermingle with erythroid islands	Aspirate smears: • Markedly decreased in number • Full-spectrum maturation • Lack of dysplastic features Core biopsy: • Markedly decreased in number • Full-spectrum maturation

Megakaryopoiesis	Aspirate smears: • Markedly decreased in number • Dysplastic features include micromegakaryocytes, forms with multiple separate nuclear lobes or forms with a single round nucleus Core biopsy: • Markedly decreased in number • Dysplastic features include micromegakaryocytes, forms with multiple separate nuclear lobes, or forms with a single round nucleus	Aspirate smears: • Markedly decreased in number • Lack of dysplastic features Core biopsy: • Markedly decreased in number • Lack of dysplastic features
PNH	Can be associated with PNH	Can be associated with PNH
Cytogenetics	Any, excluding AML-defining cytogenetics	Usually normal; lack any MDS or AML-defining abnormalities

Abbreviations: AML, acute myeloid leukemia; ANC, absolute neutrophil count; cMDS, childhood myelodysplastic syndrome; LB, low blasts; MDS, myelodysplastic syndrome; PNH, paroxysmal nocturnal hemoglobinuria; RCC, refractory cytopenia of childhood.
Adapted from references[4,8]

when present, is usually secondary to infectious causes. Splenomegaly is very rare, and hepatomegaly is usually absent.[21]

MORPHOLOGY
Peripheral Blood

In cMDS, the peripheral blood typically shows decreased numbers of platelets, white blood cells (including neutrophils), and/or red blood cells. The red blood cells usually show anisopoikilocytosis and macrocytosis with or without increased polychromasia. Neutrophils may show dysplastic features, including pseudo-Pelger-Huët nuclei, hypogranularity, and/or giant bands. Platelets may also show anisocytosis, including scattered giant forms. The proportion of blasts varies with 2% being an important threshold for classification of low blasts (<2%) versus increased/excess blasts (2%–19%).

Myelodysplastic Syndrome Without Excess Blasts (Refractory Cytopenia of Childhood / Childhood Myelodysplastic Syndrome with Low Blasts)

Approximately 80% of RCC or cMDS-LB have hypocellular marrows with cellularity that can be as low as 5% to 10% of age-appropriate normal ranges (**Fig. 1**).[24–27] Dysplasia is often, but not universally, present and can either involve at least two cell lineages or represent at least 10% in one lineage (see **Tables 1** and **2**). Dyserythropoietic features in RCC or cMDS-LB are similar to those described in adults and include abnormal nuclear segmentation (budding), multinucleation, internuclear bridges, and megaloblastoid changes. Granulocyte precursors may show nuclear hyposegmentation/pseudo-Pelger-Huët nuclei, hypo- or a-granular cytoplasm, giant bands, and nuclear-to-cytoplasmic dyssynchrony. Megakaryocytes are usually markedly decreased to absent but, when identified, are frequently small and hypolobated (micromegakaryocytes) or exhibit separated nuclear lobes.[4,8] Erythroid and megakaryocyte dysplasia are most commonly identified,[24,27] with micromegakaryocytes providing strong support for a diagnosis of RCC/cMDS-LB.

The remaining ~20% of RCC/cMDS-LB demonstrate normo- to hypercellular bone marrow, usually with a decreased myeloid-to-erythroid ratio. Erythroid precursors, especially proerythroblasts, are relatively increased. Megakaryocytes may be decreased, normal, or increased in number.[8] Dysplastic features are similar to hypocellular RCC, but >10% dysplastic forms are needed to designate megakaryocyte dysplasia in these cases.[4] At least one study has shown that RCC with multilineage dysplasia is more often normocellular or hypercellular compared with RCC without multilineage dysplasia.[24]

Core biopsies are an important and necessary component in the diagnostic workup of cMDS.[4] Overall cellularity, as well as the patchy cellular distribution typical of RCC/cMDS-LB, is best appreciated in core biopsies. RCC characteristically shows large islands of erythroid precursors (≥20 cells) with some maturational impairment and increased mitotic activity.[4,8] Some erythroid islands may abnormally localize to paratrabecular regions. Granulocytes are typically decreased with left-shifted maturation and are seen scattered throughout the marrow, including intermingled with erythroid islands. Blasts should be <5% by definition in cases of RCC/cMDS-LB. Megakaryocytes are typically decreased in hypocellular RCC/cMDS-LB but can be normal or increased in normo- to hypercellular cases.[8] Megakaryocytes may also localize abnormally to the paratrabecular regions. Micromegakaryocytes are frequent and are considered characteristic of RCC. Fibrosis is absent. As the diagnosis of RCC/cMDS-LB can be challenging, many investigators recommend two bone marrow

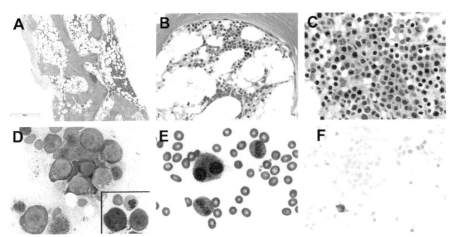

Fig. 1. RCC/cMDS-LB hypocellular. A 5 year old with mild leukopenia (WBC 4.6 K/mm³), absolute neutropenia (ANC 1150/mm³), macrocytic anemia (Hgb 10.8 g/dL; MCV 102.0 fL), and thrombocytopenia (30 K/mm³). Bone marrow evaluation showed (*A*) patchy but overall hypocellular marrow (∼10%) with large erythroid islands (Hematoxylin and eosin stain, H&E). (*B*) Erythroid islands containing > 20 cells with abnormal paratrabecular localization (H&E, 400X). (*C*) Erythroid mitotic figures (designated with red stars) (H&E, 400X). (*D*) Left-shifted erythroid maturation with both megaloblastoid and dysplastic features including nuclear budding (Wright-Giemsa, 400X). (*E*) Rare micromegakaryocytes (Wright-Giemsa, 400X). (*F*) Core biopsy CD61 immunohistochemical stain highlighting rare micromegakaryocytes (400X).

examinations at least 2 weeks apart (or from two different sites) to help establish the diagnosis.[8,26]

Myelodysplastic Syndrome, Not Otherwise Specified

Under the ICC, the category of MDS, NOS is used to classify MDS without excess blasts that do not have the typical morphologic features of RCC (**Fig. 2**).[4] This category is equivalent to the WHO category of cMDS-LB, NOS.[5] Both of these categories may lack significant cytopenias and/or dysplasia but have MDS-defining genetic abnormalities. Fibrosis can be present.

Myelodysplastic Syndrome with Increased Blasts (Myelodysplastic Syndrome with Excess Blasts / Childhood Myelodysplastic Syndrome with Increased Blasts)

MDS-EB/cMDS-IB displays similar morphologic features to RCC/cMDS-LB except for 5% to 19% blasts (**Fig. 3**).[4,5] Auer rods are not used in this classification. Unlike in adults, there are insufficient data to support making a distinction between cases with 5% to 9% bone marrow blasts and/or 2% to 4% peripheral blasts and those with 10% to 19% bone marrow blasts and/or 5% to 19% peripheral blasts.[28]

IMMUNOPHENOTYPE
Flow Cytometry

Flow cytometry is often used to aid in the diagnosis of adult MDS by identifying abnormal maturation patterns or aberrant antigen expression that suggests dysplasia.[29] Flow cytometry-based scoring systems similar to those used in adults have been applied to cMDS with variable success. Flow cytometry results are often

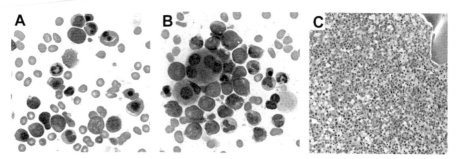

Fig. 2. MDS, NOS/cMDS-LB, NOS. A 4 year old with pancytopenia (WBC 4.4 K/mm^3, ANC 1610/mm^3, Hgb 3.3 g/dL, MCV 87.6 fL, and platelets 6 K/mm^3) and rare circulating blasts. Bone marrow evaluation showed (*A*) dysplastic erythroids with nuclear budding and irregular contours and mildly increased blasts (4.2%) (Wright-Giemsa; 400X). (*B*) Dysplastic megakaryocytes with separate nuclear lobes and/or hypolobated nuclei (Wright-Giemsa, 400X). (*C*) Hypercellular bone marrow (approaching 100%) with relatively increased erythroids but without typical RCC morphology (H&E, 200X).

normal in low-grade cMDS and the identification of immunophenotypic abnormalities among the myeloid cell populations can be difficult to interpret in pediatric patients as similar abnormalities have been identified in aplastic anemia and other pediatric cytopenias.[25,30,31] In their evaluation of 82 RCC patients, Aalbers and colleagues found that flow cytometry-based MDS scoring systems were not as applicable in RCC, as many patient samples were not cellular enough to evaluate all of the required parameters (43%).[30] In this study, only 8.5% of patients with full workups met the flow cytometry-based criteria for MDS, a markedly decreased sensitivity compared with adults.[30] In a follow-up study, Aalbers and colleagues noted several immunophenotypic findings common in RCC, including decreased CD117+ myeloblasts, promyelocytes, and immature erythroid cells; decreased granulocytes (CD33^{dim}) with a relative increase in mature CD10-positive granulocytes; increased mature lymphocytes with significantly decreased B-cell precursors (hematogones); heterogeneous expression of CD71 and CD36 on immature erythroid cells; abnormal maturation pattern of CD16 and CD13 on granulocytes; and aberrant expression of CD56 on monocytes.[25] In a small subset of patients, there was aberrant CD7 and/or CD56 expression on

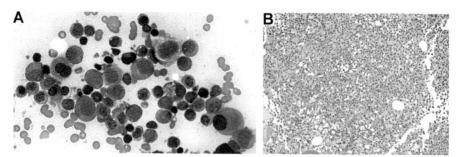

Fig. 3. MDS-EB/cMDS-IB. An 8 year old with pancytopenia (WBC 4.5 K/mm^3, ANC 1260/mm^3, Hb 9.9 g/dL, MCV 84.0 fL, and platelets 66 K/mm^3). Bone marrow evaluation showed (*A*) dysplastic megakaryocytes (small forms and a subset with mono- or hypolobated nuclei) and increased blasts (15%) (Wright-Giemsa, 400X). (*B*) Hypercellular bone marrow (~90%) (H&E, 200X). Karyotype revealed monosomy 7.

myeloblasts.[25] In addition to potential immunophenotypic alterations, approximately 37.5% to 41% of RCC patients may have identifiable paroxysmal nocturnal hemoglobinuria (PNH) clones (of variable sizes, in red cells or granulocytes) by flow cytometry.[32,33]

In higher grade MDS, flow cytometry has been shown to have more utility in children. Aalbers and colleagues demonstrated 80% (8 of 10) of cMDS with excess blasts met flow cytometry-based criteria for MDS.[30] In a follow-up study, Aalbers and colleagues identified increased CD117+ myeloblasts, promyelocytes, and erythroid cells compared with RCC, as well as aberrant CD7 expression on myeloid blasts in a subset of patients.[25] Decreased hematogones were also noted.[25,34] Other studies have confirmed that higher grade cMDS patients often demonstrate abnormal granulocytic maturation patterns and aberrant CD7 and/or CD56 antigen expression by flow cytometry.[34,35]

Immunohistochemistry

Immunohistochemical staining of bone marrow biopsies can be very helpful in diagnosing RCC/cMDS. Megakaryocytic antigens such as CD61, CD41, or CD42b enable identification of micromegakaryocytes, a finding that strongly favors a diagnosis of RCC/cMDS-LB over aplastic anemia.[4] CD34 staining may also aid in identifying increased myeloblasts. However, normal early hematogones may also express CD34, so careful marrow evaluation is required (with possible additional staining with TdT, PAX5, and/or CD79a to identify B-cell precursors). Increased myeloblasts (≥5%) by CD34 and CD117 immunostains would support a diagnosis of MDS-EB/cMDS-IB.

CYTOGENETICS

Normal karyotypes are observed in ~72% to 86% of all RCC/cMDS-LB[25,26,30,36–38] with normal karyotypes being somewhat less common in normocellular or hypercellular cases (~61%).[26] The most common cytogenetic abnormality is monosomy 7, identified in 6% to 12% of all cases,[26,30,37] but more frequently identified in normocellular or hypercellular RCC/cMDS-LB (~19%).[26] Other recurrent aberrations include trisomy 8 and complex karyotypes.[26,38] In MDS-EB/cMDS-IB, an abnormal karyotype is more commonly identified (55%–60%) with monosomy 7 being the most common abnormality (29%–32%).[36,37]

MOLECULAR FINDINGS

With the advent of NGS, many cMDS have been shown to stem from predisposing germline mutations. In some cohorts, germline mutations are identified in up to 24% to 31% of cMDS.[2,9] These germline mutations are most commonly identified in SAMD9/SAMD9L (8%) and GATA2 (7%), both of which are frequently associated with monosomy 7; in fact approximately 50% of MDS associated with monosomy 7 harbor germline mutations in these genes (**Fig. 4**).[18,39] Germline mutations in SAMD9/9L are found in both MDS with and without excess blasts, whereas germline mutations in GATA2 are more frequent in MDS-EB.[18,39] In some cases of MDS, germline mutations are identified in IBMFS genes, such as those associated with Fanconi anemia, Shwachman–Diamond syndrome, severe congenital neutropenia, and dyskeratosis congenita.[9,10,40,41]

Somatic mutations are variably identified in cMDS (9%–34%) and are more common in MDS with increased/excess blasts.[1,18,42] In RCC/cMDS-LB, somatic mutations are identified in 13% to 17% of cases, whereas in MDS-EB/cMDS-IB, somatic

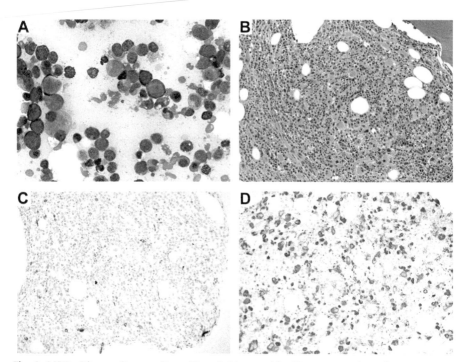

Fig. 4. MDS with germline predisposition. A 14 year old with neutropenia and severe macrocytic anemia (WBC 2.2 K/mm^3, ANC 964/mm^3, Hgb 4.4 g/dL, MCV 118.1 fL, and platelets 305 K/mm^3). Bone marrow evaluation showed (A) dysplastic megakaryocytes (separated nuclear lobes), megaloblastic erythroid precursors and mildly increased blasts (6%) (Wright-Giemsa, 400X). (B) Hypercellular bone marrow for age (70%–80%) (H&E, 200X). (C) Mildly increased blasts (CD34 immunostain, 200X). (D) Numerous megakaryocytes (CD42b immunostain, 200X). An NGS panel identified a likely pathogenic mutation in GATA2 (p.W360C, NM_032638.4:c.1080G>T) determined to be germline in origin.

mutations are identified in 65% to 68% of cases.[1,2] In addition, in patients with secondary MDS such as after chemotherapy/radiation or in those with IBMFS, somatic mutations are identified in up to 46% of cases.[42] The most commonly mutated genes include SETBP1, ASXL1, RUNX1, PTPN11, NRAS, KRAS, and NF1.[1,18,42] In total, RAS pathway mutations (most commonly PTPN11 and NRAS, but also KRAS, CBL, and NF1) are present in 12% to 45% of cases.[1,2] Cases with monosomy 7 have more somatic mutations compared with those with normal karyotypes (56% vs 18%).[1] Specifically, cases with monosomy 7 are enriched in mutations in SETBP1, ASXL1, and RUNX1, even in those without germline mutations in SAMD9/9L or GATA2.[1,18,42] Of note, genes commonly mutated in adult MDS including TET2, DNMT3A, and those involved in the spliceosome complex (such as SF3B1 and SRSF2) have not been identified in cMDS.[1,2,43]

Given the clinical and morphologic similarities between RCC/cMDS-LB and aplastic anemia, molecular studies investigating a possible autoimmune etiology for cMDS have been pursued. For example, de Vries and colleagues demonstrated skewed variability of the complementarity-determining region 3 (CDR3) length in the T-cell receptor (TCR) Vβ chains in 61% of children diagnosed with RCC, a similar percentage to the control cohort with very severe aplastic anemia (55%).[44] This finding was corroborated by a similar study showing skewed CDR3 length in 43% of RCC.[33] This skewed TCR pattern has been found to be indicative of autoimmunity in adults.[45,46] PNH clones have also been identified in cMDS (37.5%–41%), further suggesting an autoimmune/T-cell mediated etiology.[32,33] In one RCC study, de Winter and colleagues identified TCR Vβ skewing, PNH clones, or both in 61% of their RCC cohort, suggesting that a significant subset of RCC may be the result of T-cell-mediated immune dysregulation.[33]

PROGNOSIS

Like adults, pediatric patients diagnosed with MDS without excess blasts have a better prognosis when compared with those diagnosed with MDS-EB. In looking at a combined cohort of cMDS with and without excess blasts, Hasle and colleagues showed that patients with < 5% blasts (ie, without excess blasts), platelet counts of > 100 × 10^9/L, and those with favorable risk cytogenetics (ie, those with normal karyotypes, or karyotypes that included -Y, 5q-, and/or 20q and without chromosome 7 abnormalities and/or complex karyotypes) had superior survival.[20] In the cohort of MDS without excess blasts (RCC, MDS NOS, cMDS-LB), patients with normal karyotypes and/or trisomy 8 had more favorable prognoses with more stable diseases compared with those with monosomy 7.[19,21] Patients with monosomy 7 progressed to more advanced MDS at a median of 1.9 years.[21] Another favorable prognostic indicator is single lineage dysplasia when compared with multilineage dysplasia.[19] cMDS with excess blasts has a better prognosis when there is an absence of a structurally complex (≥3 chromosomal aberrations including at least one structural alteration) karyotype.[28,47] Other poor prognostic indicators include CD7 expression among the myeloid blasts and mutations in *SETBP1* (both associated with decreased overall survival).[2,34]

THERAPEUTIC OPTIONS

Three main treatment strategies exist for cMDS: watch-and-wait, immunosuppressive therapy (IST), and hematopoietic stem cell transplant (HSCT). The treatment strategy selected depends on the diagnosis (with or without excess blasts), clinical scenario, and cytogenetics. Patients with MDS, but without excess blasts (RCC/MDS, NOS/cMDS-LB), monosomy 7/del(7q), or a complex karyotype can be following with a watch-and-wait approach if the patient is relatively stable and lacks severe cytopenias (especially severe neutropenia <1000/μL), transfusion requirements, or infections.[48] For example, in one study of 65 patients with RCC, 18 of 27 patients (67%) following a watch-and-wait strategy maintained stable disease for a median of 4 to 6 years; the remaining patients developed worsening cytopenias necessitating IST and/or HSCT.[19]

   IST with cyclosporine A and anti-thymocyte globulin (ATG) has been shown to be an effective therapy in some MDS, specifically those without excess blasts, monosomy 7/del(7q), and/or complex karyotypes, particularly in the setting of hypocellular marrows.[38,48] Of note, Yoshimi and colleagues determined that IST regimens containing horse ATG had superior outcomes to IST containing rabbit ATG (74% vs 53% at 6 months).[38] In a study of 65 RCC by Hasegawa and colleagues,[19] 25 patients were initially treated with IST and another 4 were treated with IST after progression after initial monitoring. Of these 29 patients, 13 (45%) showed a response at 6 months, including 11 who remained transfusion-free. Other studies have shown a 54% to 76% IST response rate in RCC.[32,49–51] In specifically studying the association of IST response with PNH clones, Aalbers and colleagues found that patients with PNH clones (especially clones enumerated at >0.1%) had a greater likelihood of responding to IST.[32] Of note, children who receive IST remain at risk of relapse and/or clonal evolution.

Allogenic HSCT is the only curative treatment for MDS in childhood; however, due to associated morbidities, it is only used as first-line therapy for patients in which it is most effective (patients with excess blasts, monosomy 7, del(7q), and/or complex karyotypes).[48,52,53] In such cases, transplant is recommended early in the course of disease.[21,48] In studies of RCC, 61% to 74% of transplants have led to remission, with secondary graft failures occurring in 5% to 17% of patients and treatment-related mortality ranging from 9% to 32%.[19,21,49] In studies of MDS-EB, transplant has been found to have an event-free survival of 61% to 64%, with therapy-related mortality ranging from 14% to 23%.[28,52]

DIFFERENTIAL DIAGNOSIS

The differential diagnosis for cMDS without increased blasts, particularly hypocellular cases, is quite broad. Nonneoplastic entities including viral infections (such as cytomegalovirus, herpesvirus, Epstein–Barr virus, and parvovirus B19), nutritional deficiencies (including vitamin B12, folate, and vitamin E), metabolic disorders (such as mevalonate kinase deficiency), autoimmune and rheumatological diseases (including systemic lupus erythematosus and autoimmune lymphoproliferative disorder), and mitochondrial deletions (such as Pearson syndrome) can lead to dysplastic features in children that mimic RCC/cMDS-LB.[8] Given that RCC and cMDS-LB are often hypocellular, the differential diagnosis also includes aplastic anemia. However, there are distinctive features of RCC/cMDS-LB that can help differentiate hypocellular MDS from aplastic anemia, including the presence of increased and enlarged erythroid islands, left-shifted erythroid maturation, and dysplasia (most notably micromegakaryocytes) (see **Table 2**). In studies from the European Working Group of MDS in Childhood, most RCC could be differentiated from severe aplastic anemia by morphology alone with a concordance rate of 76%,[54] though other groups have shown less concordance (~53%).[55] It is notable that in aplastic anemia treated with IST, subsequent morphologic distinction between aplastic anemia and RCC/cMDS-LB can be extremely challenging.[26]

At initial presentation, IBMFS can have the bone marrow morphology of RCC/cMDS-LB.[26] Such IBMFS include Fanconi anemia, dyskeratosis congenita, Shwachman–Diamond syndrome, severe congenital neutropenia, and Diamond–Blackfan anemia.[10,40,41,56] In particular, in Fanconi anemia, it can be challenging to determine whether morphologic changes are due to the germline mutation itself or the result of subsequent MDS development; therefore, classifications specific to patients with Fanconi anemia have been proposed.[57]

Other germline mutations such as those in GATA2, RUNX1, and SAMD9/SAMD9L can also present as RCC/cMDS-LB or MDS-EB/cMDS-IB.[10,18,39,58,59] Per the WHO, some cMDS-LB represent dysplastic progression of IBMFS or genetic germline predisposition syndromes, further complicating the diagnosis. Therefore, careful attention to clinical and family history, physical examination findings (for physical anomalies), and other laboratory values is needed to help differentiate many of these cases. Consideration of molecular testing may be warranted, even in the absence of characteristic features, to identify de novo germline mutations.[10,59] In cases which progress to a higher grade MDS with increased/excess blasts, it may be appropriate to classify based on their germline predisposition syndrome [myeloid neoplasms with germline predisposition (WHO)[5] or hematologic neoplasms with germline predisposition (ICC)][3,4] depending on the clinical scenario.

Under the new ICC and WHO classifications of hematopoietic neoplasms, the percentage of blasts required to diagnose AML with defining genetic fusions and/ or mutations was decreased from $\geq$20% to $\geq$10% (ICC) or any blast count (WHO).[3,5] Therefore, in pediatric patients diagnosed with MDS, such recurrent fusions or mutations (such as NPM1) may necessitate a diagnosis of (and treatment for) AML.

In certain settings, juvenile myelomonocytic leukemia (JMML) and myeloid leukemia associated with Down syndrome (ML-DS) may also be included in the differential diagnosis. In JMML, the bone marrow is usually hypercellular with myeloid hyperplasia and less than 20% blasts; erythroid hyperplasia may also be present. However, dysplasia is usually not a prominent feature.[60] In contrast to MDS, JMML usually presents with peripheral monocytosis, leukocytosis, and splenomegaly, all typically absent in MDS. Both JMML and ML-DS more commonly occur in children under 5 years of age.[60,61] As its name implies, ML-DS occurs in children with Down syndrome but can also occur in patients who are mosaic for trisomy 21 and hence may not show typical clinical features. ML-DS can present as an MDS with< 20% blasts (typically with megakaryocytic differentiation), megakaryocyte hyperplasia and dysplasia, and often increased fibrosis.

SUMMARY

In summary, cMDS is a rare diagnosis requiring the incorporation of peripheral blood, bone marrow, cytogenetics, and molecular results, as well as the exclusion of nonneoplastic etiologies that may cause dysplasia. With the expansion of molecular testing, increased numbers of patients have been shown to have germline predisposition due to IBMFS or mutations in other genes predisposing to hematologic neoplasms such as GATA2, RUNX1, and SAMD9/SAMD9L. In contrast to adults, cMDS has a different biological signature, often containing somatic RAS pathway or SETBP1, ASXL1, and/or RUNX1 mutations. Correlation of the clinical findings, blast percentage, karyotype, and molecular results helps to guide treatment, whether it is a watch-and-wait strategy, treatment with IST, or an HSCT.

CLINICS CARE POINTS

- Childhood myelodysplastic syndrome (cMDS) is divided into two main categories: (1) refractory cytopenia of childhood/MDS with low blasts for cases with <2% peripheral blood and <5% bone marrow blasts and (2) MDS-excess blasts/MDS-increased blasts for cases with $\geq$2% peripheral blood or $\geq$5% bone marrow blasts.
- The diagnosis of cMDS requires clinical and pathologic correlation, including integration of peripheral blood features, bone marrow aspirate and biopsy findings, and cytogenetics results. The diagnosis is often challenging and may require multiple bone marrow evaluations for final classification.
- Molecular testing is clinical useful, commonly identifies somatic RAS pathway mutations, and can alter treatment if an underlying germline mutations is present.
- The differential diagnosis for cMDS is broad and includes nonneoplastic entities, such as infections, nutritional deficiencies, and metabolic disorders.

DISCLOSURE

The authors have nothing to disclose.

REFERENCES

1. Pastor V, Hirabayashi S, Karow A, et al. Mutational landscape in children with myelodysplastic syndromes is distinct from adults: specific somatic drivers and novel germline variants. Leukemia 2017;31(3):759–62.
2. Schwartz JR, Ma J, Lamprecht T, et al. The genomic landscape of pediatric myelodysplastic syndromes. Nat Commun 2017;8(1):1557.
3. Arber DA, Orazi A, Hasserjian RP, et al. International Consensus classification of myeloid neoplasms and acute leukemias: integrating morphologic, clinical, and genomic data. Blood 2022;140(11):1200–28.
4. Rudelius M, Weinberg OK, Niemeyer CM, et al. The International Consensus Classification (ICC) of hematologic neoplasms with germline predisposition, pediatric myelodysplastic syndrome, and juvenile myelomonocytic leukemia. Virchows Arch 2023;482(1):113–30.
5. Khoury JD, Solary E, Abla O, et al. The 5th edition of the World Health organization classification of haematolymphoid tumours: myeloid and histiocytic/dendritic neoplasms. Leukemia 2022;36(7):1703–19.
6. Hasle H, Niemeyer CM, Chessells JM, et al. A pediatric approach to the WHO classification of myelodysplastic and myeloproliferative diseases. Leukemia 2003;17(2):277–82.
7. Baumann I, Niemeyer CM, Bennett JM, et al. Childhood myelodysplastic syndrome. In: Swerdlow SH, Campo E, Harris NL, et al, editors. WHO Classification of tumours of haematopoietic and lymphoid tissues. Lyon, France: International Agency for Research on Cancer; 2008. p. 104–7.
8. Baumann I, Niemeyer CM, Bennett JM. Childhood myelodysplastic syndrome. In: Swerdlow SH, Campo E, Harris NL, et al, editors. WHO classification of tumours of haematopoietic and lymphoid tissues. Lyon, France: International Agency for Research on Cancer; 2017. p. 116–20.
9. Keel SB, Scott A, Sanchez-Bonilla M, et al. Genetic features of myelodysplastic syndrome and aplastic anemia in pediatric and young adult patients. Haematologica 2016;101(11):1343–50.
10. Kennedy AL, Shimamura A. Genetic predisposition to MDS: clinical features and clonal evolution. Blood 2019;133(10):1071–85.
11. Passmore SJ, Chessells JM, Kempski H, et al. Paediatric myelodysplastic syndromes and juvenile myelomonocytic leukaemia in the UK: a population-based study of incidence and survival. Br J Haematol 2003;121(5):758–67.
12. Bhatia S, Krailo MD, Chen Z, et al. Therapy-related myelodysplasia and acute myeloid leukemia after Ewing sarcoma and primitive neuroectodermal tumor of bone: a report from the Children's Oncology Group. Blood 2007;109(1):46–51.
13. Kushner BH, Cheung NK, Kramer K, et al. Neuroblastoma and treatment-related myelodysplasia/leukemia: the Memorial Sloan-Kettering experience and a literature review. J Clin Oncol 1998;16(12):3880–9.
14. Bhatia S, Sather HN, Pabustan OB, et al. Low incidence of second neoplasms among children diagnosed with acute lymphoblastic leukemia after 1983. Blood 2002;99(12):4257–64.
15. Schmiegelow K, Al-Modhwahi I, Andersen MK, et al. Methotrexate/6-mercaptopurine maintenance therapy influences the risk of a second malignant neoplasm after childhood acute lymphoblastic leukemia: results from the NOPHO ALL-92 study. Blood 2009;113(24):6077–84.
16. Hasle H, Kerndrup G, Jacobsen BB. Childhood myelodysplastic syndrome in Denmark: incidence and predisposing conditions. Leukemia 1995;9(9):1569–72.

17. Hasle H, Wadsworth LD, Massing BG, et al. A population-based study of childhood myelodysplastic syndrome in British Columbia, Canada. Br J Haematol 1999;106(4):1027–32.

18. Sahoo SS, Pastor VB, Goodings C, et al. Clinical evolution, genetic landscape and trajectories of clonal hematopoiesis in SAMD9/SAMD9L syndromes. Nat Med 2021;27(10):1806–17.

19. Hasegawa D, Chen X, Hirabayashi S, et al. Clinical characteristics and treatment outcome in 65 cases with refractory cytopenia of childhood defined according to the WHO 2008 classification. Br J Haematol 2014;166(5):758–66.

20. Hasle H, Baumann I, Bergstrasser E, et al. The International Prognostic Scoring System (IPSS) for childhood myelodysplastic syndrome (MDS) and juvenile myelomonocytic leukemia (JMML). Leukemia 2004;18(12):2008–14.

21. Kardos G, Baumann I, Passmore SJ, et al. Refractory anemia in childhood: a retrospective analysis of 67 patients with particular reference to monosomy 7. Blood 2003;102(6):1997–2003.

22. Luna-Fineman S, Shannon KM, Atwater SK, et al. Myelodysplastic and myeloproliferative disorders of childhood: a study of 167 patients. Blood 1999;93(2):459–66.

23. Sasaki H, Manabe A, Kojima S, et al. Myelodysplastic syndrome in childhood: a retrospective study of 189 patients in Japan. Leukemia 2001;15(11):1713–20.

24. Iwafuchi H, Ito M. Differences in the bone marrow histology between childhood myelodysplastic syndrome with multilineage dysplasia and refractory cytopenia of childhood without multilineage dysplasia. Histopathology 2019;74(2):239–47.

25. Aalbers AM, van den Heuvel-Eibrink MM, Baumann I, et al. Bone marrow immunophenotyping by flow cytometry in refractory cytopenia of childhood. Haematologica 2015;100(3):315–23.

26. Niemeyer CM, Baumann I. Classification of childhood aplastic anemia and myelodysplastic syndrome. Hematology Am Soc Hematol Educ Program 2011;2011:84–9.

27. Polychronopoulou S, Panagiotou JP, Kossiva L, et al. Clinical and morphological features of paediatric myelodysplastic syndromes: a review of 34 cases. Acta Paediatr 2004;93(8):1015–23.

28. Kikuchi A, Hasegawa D, Ohtsuka Y, et al. Outcome of children with refractory anaemia with excess of blast (RAEB) and RAEB in transformation (RAEB-T) in the Japanese MDS99 study. Br J Haematol 2012;158(5):657–61.

29. Westers TM, Ireland R, Kern W, et al. Standardization of flow cytometry in myelodysplastic syndromes: a report from an international consortium and the European LeukemiaNet Working Group. Leukemia 2012;26(7):1730–41.

30. Aalbers AM, van den Heuvel-Eibrink MM, de Haas V, et al. Applicability of a reproducible flow cytometry scoring system in the diagnosis of refractory cytopenia of childhood. Leukemia 2013;27(9):1923–5.

31. Chisholm KM, Xu M, Davis B, et al. Evaluation of the utility of bone marrow morphology and ancillary studies in pediatric patients under surveillance for myelodysplastic syndrome. Am J Clin Pathol 2018;149(6):499–513.

32. Aalbers AM, van der Velden VH, Yoshimi A, et al. The clinical relevance of minor paroxysmal nocturnal hemoglobinuria clones in refractory cytopenia of childhood: a prospective study by EWOG-MDS. Leukemia 2014;28(1):189–92.

33. de Winter DTC, Langerak AW, Te Marvelde J, et al. The variable biological signature of refractory cytopenia of childhood (RCC), a retrospective EWOG-MDS study. Leuk Res 2021;108:106652.

34. Veltroni M, Sainati L, Zecca M, et al. Advanced pediatric myelodysplastic syndromes: can immunophenotypic characterization of blast cells be a diagnostic and prognostic tool? Pediatr Blood Cancer 2009;52(3):357–63.
35. Oliveira AF, Tansini A, Vidal DO, et al. Characteristics of the phenotypic abnormalities of bone marrow cells in childhood myelodysplastic syndromes and juvenile myelomonocytic leukemia, Pediatr Blood Cancer, 64 (4), 2017, e26285.
36. Niemeyer CM, Kratz CP. Paediatric myelodysplastic syndromes and juvenile myelomonocytic leukaemia: molecular classification and treatment options. Br J Haematol 2008;140(6):610–24.
37. Pui CH, Schrappe M, Ribeiro RC, et al. Childhood and adolescent lymphoid and myeloid leukemia. Hematology Am Soc Hematol Educ Program 2004;118–45.
38. Yoshimi A, van den Heuvel-Eibrink MM, Baumann I, et al. Comparison of horse and rabbit antithymocyte globulin in immunosuppressive therapy for refractory cytopenia of childhood. Haematologica 2014;99(4):656–63.
39. Wlodarski MW, Hirabayashi S, Pastor V, et al. Prevalence, clinical characteristics, and prognosis of GATA2-related myelodysplastic syndromes in children and adolescents. Blood 2016;127(11):1387–97 ; quiz 1518.
40. Cada M, Segbefia CI, Klaassen R, et al. The impact of category, cytopathology and cytogenetics on development and progression of clonal and malignant myeloid transformation in inherited bone marrow failure syndromes. Haematologica 2015;100(5):633–42.
41. Yoshimi A, Niemeyer C, Baumann I, et al. High incidence of Fanconi anaemia in patients with a morphological picture consistent with refractory cytopenia of childhood. Br J Haematol 2013;160(1):109–11.
42. Kozyra EJ, Hirabayashi S, Bengt Pastor Loyola V, et al. Clonal mutational landscape of childhood myelodysplastic syndromes. Blood 2015;126(23):1662.
43. Hirabayashi S, Flotho C, Moetter J, et al. Spliceosomal gene aberrations are rare, coexist with oncogenic mutations, and are unlikely to exert a driver effect in childhood MDS and JMML. Blood 2012;119(11):e96–9.
44. de Vries AC, Langerak AW, Verhaaf B, et al. T-cell receptor Vbeta CDR3 oligoclonality frequently occurs in childhood refractory cytopenia (MDS-RC) and severe aplastic anemia. Leukemia 2008;22(6):1170–4.
45. Kook H, Risitano AM, Zeng W, et al. Changes in T-cell receptor VB repertoire in aplastic anemia: effects of different immunosuppressive regimens. Blood 2002; 99(10):3668–75.
46. Risitano AM, Kook H, Zeng W, et al. Oligoclonal and polyclonal CD4 and CD8 lymphocytes in aplastic anemia and paroxysmal nocturnal hemoglobinuria measured by V beta CDR3 spectratyping and flow cytometry. Blood 2002; 100(1):178–83.
47. Gohring G, Michalova K, Beverloo HB, et al. Complex karyotype newly defined: the strongest prognostic factor in advanced childhood myelodysplastic syndrome. Blood 2010;116(19):3766–9.
48. Locatelli F, Strahm B. How I treat myelodysplastic syndromes of childhood. Blood 2018;131(13):1406–14.
49. Hama A, Hasegawa D, Manabe A, et al. Prospective validation of the provisional entity of refractory cytopenia of childhood, proposed by the World Health Organization. Br J Haematol 2022;196(4):1031–9.
50. Hama A, Takahashi Y, Muramatsu H, et al. Comparison of long-term outcomes between children with aplastic anemia and refractory cytopenia of childhood who received immunosuppressive therapy with antithymocyte globulin and cyclosporine. Haematologica 2015;100(11):1426–33.

51. Yoshimi A, Baumann I, Fuhrer M, et al. Immunosuppressive therapy with anti-thymocyte globulin and cyclosporine A in selected children with hypoplastic refractory cytopenia. Haematologica 2007;92(3):397–400.
52. Strahm B, Nollke P, Zecca M, et al. Hematopoietic stem cell transplantation for advanced myelodysplastic syndrome in children: results of the EWOG-MDS 98 study. Leukemia 2011;25(3):455–62.
53. Trobaugh-Lotrario AD, Kletzel M, Quinones RR, et al. Monosomy 7 associated with pediatric acute myeloid leukemia (AML) and myelodysplastic syndrome (MDS): successful management by allogeneic hematopoietic stem cell transplant (HSCT). Bone Marrow Transplant 2005;35(2):143–9.
54. Baumann I, Fuhrer M, Behrendt S, et al. Morphological differentiation of severe aplastic anaemia from hypocellular refractory cytopenia of childhood: reproducibility of histopathological diagnostic criteria. Histopathology 2012;61(1):10–7.
55. Forester CM, Sartain SE, Guo D, et al. Pediatric aplastic anemia and refractory cytopenia: a retrospective analysis assessing outcomes and histomorphologic predictors. Am J Hematol 2015;90(4):320–6.
56. Niemeyer CM, Baumann I. Myelodysplastic syndrome in children and adolescents. Semin Hematol 2008;45(1):60–70.
57. Behrens YL, Gohring G, Bawadi R, et al. A novel classification of hematologic conditions in patients with Fanconi anemia. Haematologica 2021;106(11):3000–3.
58. Churpek JE, Pyrtel K, Kanchi KL, et al. Genomic analysis of germ line and somatic variants in familial myelodysplasia/acute myeloid leukemia. Blood 2015;126(22):2484–90.
59. Zhang MY, Keel SB, Walsh T, et al. Genomic analysis of bone marrow failure and myelodysplastic syndromes reveals phenotypic and diagnostic complexity. Haematologica 2015;100(1):42–8.
60. Baumann I, Bennett JM, Niemeyer CM, et al. Juvenile myelomonocytic leukaemia. In: Swerdlow SH, Campo E, Harris NL, et al, editors. WHO classification of tumours of haematopoietic and lymphoid tissues. Lyon, France: International Agency for Research on Cancer; 2017. p. 89–92.
61. Arber DA, Baumann I, Niemeyer CM, et al. Myeloid proliferations associated with Down syndrome. In: Swerdlow SH, Campo E, Harris NL, et al, editors. WHO classification of tumours of haematopoietic and lymphoid tissues. Lyon, France: International Agency for Research on Cancer; 2017. p. 169–71.

Acute Myeloid Leukemia Arising from Myelodysplastic Syndromes

Adelaide Kwon, MD, Olga K. Weinberg, MD*

KEYWORDS

- Acute myeloid leukemia • Myelodysplastic syndrome • Genomics • Progression
- Outcome

KEY POINTS

- Myelodysplastic neoplasms are a group of clonal hematopoietic bone marrow disorders with an increased risk of transformation to acute myeloid leukemia (AML).
- De novo AML results from an inciting genomic event that leads to expansion of the leukemic clone, whereas AML arising from MDS typically evolves in a stepwise fashion with multiple hits accumulating over time and tend to exhibit more mutated genes than do those with de novo AML.
- Mutations in *SRSF2*, *SF3B1*, *U2AF1*, *ZRSR2*, *ASXL1*, *EZH2*, *BCOR*, *RUNX1*, and *STAG2* are highly specific for secondary AML and are now included in both the World Health Organization and the International Consensus Classification updated classification of AML arising from MDS.

INTRODUCTION AND HISTORY

Myelodysplastic syndromes (MDS), also known as myelodysplastic neoplasms, are a group of clonal hematopoietic bone marrow disorders with an increased risk of transformation to acute myeloid leukemia (AML).[1,2] MDS is characterized by dysplasia in the myeloid lineages and ineffective hematopoiesis and, although a distinct entity, often forms a spectrum with AML.[1–3] The progression to AML from MDS is not uncommon but more likely to occur in subtypes with increased myeloblasts and less likely to occur in subtypes with prolonged, indolent, progressive bone marrow failure.[1–5] AML arising from MDS has a worse prognosis, remission rate, and rate of survival compared with de novo AML.[6,7] Historically, the distinction between diagnosing MDS or AML has been based on blast count.[8–11] However, recent advancements in next-generation sequencing have shifted diagnostic criteria toward a greater emphasis on genetic features over strict blast cutoffs.[1,2]

Department of Pathology, University of Texas Southwestern Medical Center, Dallas, TX, USA
* Corresponding author.
E-mail address: olga.weinberg@utsouthwestern.edu

Clin Lab Med 43 (2023) 657–667
https://doi.org/10.1016/j.cll.2023.07.001
0272-2712/23/© 2023 Elsevier Inc. All rights reserved.

labmed.theclinics.com

In 1976, the first French-American-British (FAB) classifications were established and published, defining 30% as the blast cutoff between MDS and AML, with less than 30% blasts classified as MDS and greater than or equal to 30% blasts classified as AML.[8,9] MDS was further divided into 5 subtypes. Although refractory anemia with ring sideroblasts and chronic myelomonocytic leukemia were characterized by the presence of ringed sideroblasts and excess monocytes, respectively, the other 3 subtypes were exclusively defined by the percentage of blasts seen in the peripheral blood and bone marrow.[8] Refractory anemia (RA) was defined by less than or equal to 1% blasts in the peripheral blood and less than 5% in the bone marrow, refractory anemia with excess blasts (RAEB) was defined by less than 5% blasts in the peripheral blood and 5% to 20% in the bone marrow, and RAEB in transformation (RAEB-T) was defined by greater than or equal to 5% blasts in the peripheral blood and 21% to 29% in the bone marrow.[8,12,13] As to be expected, MDS subtypes with higher blast percentages were also noted to have a higher risk of transformation to AML and poorer prognosis.[12–14]

The 30% blast cutoff was somewhat controversially changed to 20% with the establishment of the World Health Organization (WHO) classification of hematolymphoid tumours guidelines in 2001, effectively excluding RAEB-T patients from MDS and instead reclassifying them as AML.[10,15] The rationale for this decision was that although MDS cases did not always progress to AML, patients with MDS with greater than 20% blasts had a similar treatment response compared with patients with AML.[10,15] However, a concern arose that merging RAEB-T and AML would lead to the loss of distinction between the more indolent pace, distinct morphologic dysplasia, and poor response to chemotherapy of MDS in comparison to AML in these patients.[16] Despite these concerns, the new threshold remained. RAEB was kept as a separate MDS subcategory but was further subdivided into RAEB-1 and RAEB-2, defined as blasts making up 5% to -9% of the cells in the bone marrow and blasts making up 10% to 19% of the cells in the bone marrow, respectively.[10,15] In the 2008 update to the WHO guidelines, these subcategories were further expanded to account for peripheral blood blast count, with RAEB-1 including cases with 2% to -4% blasts in the peripheral blood and RAEB-2 including cases with 5% to 19% blasts in the peripheral blood.[11] RAEB was later renamed in the 2016 update to the WHO guidelines to MDS with excess blasts (MDS-EB), with RAEB-1 and RAEB-2 renamed as MDS-EB1 and MDS-EB2, although the blast count criteria remained the same.[17]

In recent years, advancements in the field of genetics and next-generation sequencing technology have led to a better understanding of the genetic features that distinguish MDS and AML, and this has led to a shift in focus away from the traditional morphologic features and blast count cutoffs in categorizing MDS and AML to a more genetic- and molecular-based approach.[1,2] The recently released fifth edition of the WHO guidelines as well as the new International Consensus Classification (ICC) guidelines, both published in 2022, have redefined these blast cutoffs to be less rigid, allowing for more flexibility with diagnoses and treatment strategies.[1,2]

INCIDENCE

The incidence of MDS per year is approximately 3.6 cases per 100,000, and the incidence of AML per year is approximately 4.1 per 100,000.[18] Approximately 25% to 35% of AML cases are secondary, and approximately 60% to 80% of secondary AML are from MDS; this makes AML arising from MDS approximately 15% to 28% of AML cases.[6,19–21] Approximately 30% of MDS cases become AML.[6,19,20] Subtypes that have increased blasts are more likely to undergo this transformation, whereas more indolent subtypes with progressive bone marrow failure are less likely to transform into AML.

MORPHOLOGIC FEATURES

Morphologically, MDS is characterized by cytopenia and myeloid lineage dysplasia.[1,2] In contrast, although some subcategories of AML, including AML, myelodysplasia-related (AML-MR), also demonstrate dysplastic features, not all types of AML do so.[1,2] Dysplastic features found in both MDS and AML-MR include very small or abnormally lobated megakaryocytes (**Fig. 1**A); nuclear budding, irregular nuclear borders (**Fig. 1**B), multinucleation, megaloblastosis, karyorrhexis, ring sideroblasts (**Fig. 1**C), or cytoplasmic vacuoles in erythroid precursors; and hypogranular (**Fig. 1**D), hyposegmented, or bizarrely segmented neutrophils.[1,2] Although the distinction between these 2 entities has historically then fallen to blast count, the fifth edition of the WHO and the new ICC guidelines propose a greater emphasis on genetic features, allowing for more flexibility and individualization with patient treatment.[1,2]

The 2022 WHO guidelines broadly categorize MDS into 2 groups: MDS with defining genetic abnormalities and MDS, morphologically defined, with genetic features outweighing morphologic features.[1] MDS with defining genetic abnormalities include MDS with low blasts and isolated 5q deletion (MDS-5q), MDS with low blasts and *SF3B1* mutation (MDS-*SF3B1*), and MDS with biallelic *TP53* inactivation (MDS-bi*TP53*).[1] Morphologically defined MDS includes MDS with low blasts; MDS, hypoplastic, a newly distinct disease entity; and MDS with increased blasts, which replaces

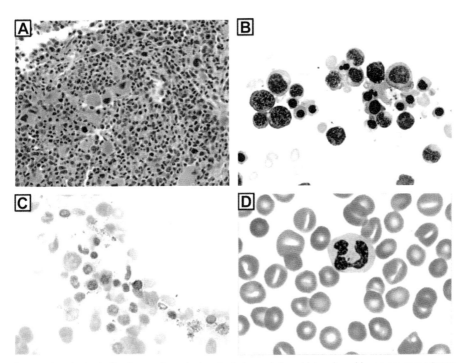

Fig. 1. Morphologic findings of myelodysplasia in peripheral blood and bone marrow. Bone marrow biopsy with megakaryocytes demonstrating small size and hypolobation (*A*). Bone marrow aspirate smears with erythroid precursors demonstrating nuclear budding, irregular nuclear borders (*B*), and ring sideroblasts (*C*). Peripheral blood smear with a segmented neutrophil demonstrating hypogranulation (*D*). [Hematoxylin and eosin stain in (*A*) (20x objective), Wright-Giemsa stains in images (*B*, *D*) (100x objective), and iron stain in (*C*) (100x objective)].

MDS-EB but otherwise retains the same definitions and blast cutoffs.[1] Similarly, AML is broadly categorized into AML with defining genetic abnormalities and AML defined by differentiation.[1] Defining genetic abnormalities include *PML::RARA* fusion, *RUNX1::RUNX1T1* fusion, *CBFB::MYH11* fusion, *DEK::NUP214* fusion, *RBM15::MRTFA* fusion, *BCR::ABL1* fusion, *KMT2A* rearrangement, *MECOM* rearrangement, *NUP98* rearrangement, *NPM1* mutation, and *CEBPA* mutation.[1] Key to this AML family is the removal of the 20% blast requirement for diagnosis for all but AML with *BCR::ABL1* and AML with *CEBPA* mutation.[1] AML with defining genetic abnormalities also includes AML-MR as well as an entity for AML with other defined genetic alterations to cover rare or newly emerging diseases.[1] On the other hand, cases of AML defined by differentiation lack defining genetic alterations and are classified based on maturation and morphology instead. The entities in this AML family include AML with minimal differentiation, AML with without maturation, AML with maturation, acute basophilic leukemia, acute myelomonocytic leukemia, acute monocytic leukemia, acute erythroid leukemia, and acute megakaryoblastic leukemia.[1] Although the blast cutoff for these cases remains greater than or equal to 20% and, similarly, the blast cutoff differentiating MDS (MDS-IB2) from AML remains 20%, there is a clear shift in focus to genetic abnormalities with the elimination of blast cutoffs in AML with defining genetic abnormalities and a general agreement that MDS-IB2 can be treated as equivalent to AML from a therapeutic or clinical trial standpoint.[1,22]

The 2022 ICC guidelines identify many of the same defining genetic abnormalities for MDS and AML as the WHO guidelines and continue to emphasize these genetic features in diagnosis, but the ICC guidelines elect to approach the blast cutoff differently. MDS entities in this classification include MDS with mutated *SF3B1*; MDS with del(5q); MDS with mutated *TP53*; MDS, not otherwise specified (MDS); MDS with excess blasts; and MDS/AML, a newly defined category to cover entities with bone marrow or peripheral blood blast counts between 10% and 19%. On the other hand, AML-defining genetic abnormalities include *PML::RARA*, other *RARA* rearrangements, *RUNX1::RUNX1T1*, *CBFB::MYH11*, *MLLT3::KMT2A*, other *KMT2A* rearrangements, *DEK::NUP214*, *GATA2*, *MECOM(EVI1)*, other *MECOM* rearrangements, *BCR::ABL1*, *NPM1* mutations, in-frame bZIP *CEBPA* mutations, *TP53* mutations, and other rare recurring translocations.[2] Unlike how the WHO guidelines eliminated blast cutoffs entirely when classifying AML with these defining genetic abnormalities, the ICC guidelines use greater than 10% as the blast cutoff required for diagnosis.[2] However, in cases without these defining abnormalities and in differentiating between MDS and AML, while the WHO guidelines elected to retain the 20% blast cutoff, the ICC guidelines instead define a new entity, MDS/AML, for cases with blast counts between 10% and 19%.[2] With the understanding that these cases should be treated as either MDS or AML on an individual basis, the establishment of the MDS/AML entity effectively lowers the AML blast threshold to 10% from a therapeutic or clinical trial standpoint.

GENETIC AND MOLECULAR FEATURES

As discussed earlier, the 2022 WHO and ICC guidelines highly emphasize the genetic features distinguishing MDS and AML and update these definitions to account for advancements in the understanding of the molecular and genetic profiles of these entities. There is significant overlap between the genetic abnormalities identified as AML-defining in the 2022 WHO and ICC classifications, though some differences remain. In both classifications, the presence of these mutations is enough to diagnose AML at blast percentages lower than 20%, with the mutations alone enough for diagnosis in the WHO guidelines and a blast cutoff of 10% enough in the ICC guidelines.[1,2] Although the blast cutoff for diagnosing AML instead of MDS in cases without defining genetic alterations remains 20% in the WHO guidelines, it is suggested that MDS-IB2 can be considered AML-equivalent in treatment and clinical practice, making the delineation between the 2 entities less rigid at higher blast percentages.[1] The WHO guidelines have also made several updates to the former entity AML with myelodysplasia-related changes, which has now been redesignated AML, myelodysplasia-related (AML-MR). These changes similarly shift focus away from strict morphologic features for diagnosis to a more molecular- and genetic-based approach by introducing mutation-based definitions and updating defining cytogenetic criteria.[1] Likewise, the ICC guidelines have defined a new entity, MDS/AML, to cover cases in the 10% to 19% blast count window, with a similar focus on identification of specific gene mutations and cytogenetic abnormalities.[2]

Both the WHO and ICC have identified 8 genes associated with myelodysplasia: ASXL1, EZH2, BCOR, SF3B1, SRSF2, U2AF1, ZRSR2, and STAG2.[1,2] The ICC also identifies RUNX1 as a myelodysplasia-related genetic mutation.[2] **Table 1** showcases the differences between these 2 classification systems. These 8 genes have greater than 95% specificity for AML with myelodysplasia compared with de novo AML and are involved in histone modification (ASXL1, BCOR, EZH2), spliceosomes (SF3B1, SRSF2, ZRSR2, U2AF1), and the cohesin complex (STAG2), whereas RUNX1 is a transcription factor mutation.[3,23–26] SF3B1 in particular has long been associated with the development of ring sideroblasts; inhibition and knock out studies in vitro and with mouse models have demonstrated a causative relationship, and an increased variant

Table 1
Differences in 2022 WHO and ICC myelodysplasia-defining abnormalities

2022 WHO	ICC
Defining cytogenetic abnormalities	
ASXL1	ASXL1
EZH2	EZH2
BCOR	BCOR
SF3B1	SF3B1
SRSF2	SRSF2
U2AF1	U2AF1
ZRSR2	ZRSR2
STAG2	STAG2
	RUNX1
Defining somatic mutations	
Complex karyotype (≥3 abnormalities)	Complex karyotype (≥3 abnormalities)
5q deletion or loss	5q deletion or loss
Monosomy 7, 7q deletion, or loss	Monosomy 7, 7q deletion, or loss
11q deletion	Trisomy 8
12p deletion or loss	11q deletion
Monosomy 13 or 13q deletion	12p deletion or loss
17p deletion or loss	17p deletion or loss
Isochromosome 17q	Isochromosome 17q
Isodicentric X chromosome with Xq13 breakpoint	20q deletion
	Isodicentric X chromosome with Xq13 breakpoint

allele frequency (VAF) correlates with a higher percentage of ring sideroblasts.[3,26–28] Other studies have demonstrated that the frequency and distribution of genetic mutations differs on the spectrum of myelodysplasia and suggest that additional mutations progressively drive the transformation of clonal hematopoiesis of indeterminate potential (CHIP) to MDS to MDS/AML and AML-MR.[19,23,29–33] For example, mutations in *TP53*, *DNMT3A*, *TET2*, and *ASXL1*, epigenetic modifiers, are found in all 3 entities, suggesting that these mutations occur early in the disease process, whereas mutations in transcription factors such as *RUNX1* and *GATA2* are more commonly seen in MDS, MDS/AML, and AML-MR, suggesting that these mutations occur later in the advancement from CHIP to more aggressive entities.[19,23,29,34,35] Finally, mutations in other transcription factors and activating signaling genes such as *CEBPA*, *FLT3*, and *NRAS* are commonly seen in MDS/AML and AML-MR, suggesting that the acquisition of these mutations may play a role in driving MDS transformation to AML.[19,23,24,29] **Table 2** showcases some of these commonly mutated genes.

TP53 alterations occur in 5% to 10% of de novo MDS or AML cases and 20% to 40% of therapy-related myeloid neoplasms.[36] *TP53* alteration include mutations, cytogenetic abnormalities leading to the physical loss of a *TP53* gene or copy-neutral loss of heterozygosity (cn-LOH) of chromosome 17p. ICC introduced a new category termed "myeloid neoplasms with mutated *TP53*" that groups together 3 disease entities with similar aggressive clinical biology that warrants a unified therapeutic approach. The 3 entities within this broad category are MDS with mutated *TP53*, MDS/AML with mutated *TP53,* and AML with mutated *TP53*, separated by different bone marrow blast percentages as well as the degree of *TP53* mutational burden. The blast percentage criteria for the *TP53*-mutated entities are 0% to 9% for MDS, 10% to 19% for MDS/AML, and greater than or equal to 20% for AML.[2] In the classification hierarchy, MDS with mutated *TP53* category supersedes MDS-EB1 and the MDS/AML category supersedes MDS-EB2. In addition, pure erythroid leukemia, which is highly associated with *TP53* mutations, is now included under AML with mutated *TP53* and is mostly eliminated as an entity by the ICC. "Multi-hit" mutational status is required for a diagnosis of *TP53*-mutated MDS, because monoallelic *TP53* mutations have a less deleterious effect on biology and prognosis. "Multi-hit" is defined by the presence of 2 or more distinct *TP53* mutations with VAF greater than or equal to 10% or a single *TP53* mutation associated with either a cytogenetic deletion involving the *TP53* locus at 17p13.1[2]; a VAF of greater than 50%; or[3] cn-LOH at the 17p *TP53* locus. In the absence of LOH information, the presence of a single *TP53* mutation in the context of any complex karyotype is considered equivalent to a multi-hit *TP53*. By contrast, any (monoallelic or otherwise) somatic mutation of *TP53* with a

Table 2
Common mutations in the progression from clonal hematopoiesis of indeterminate potential to myelodysplastic syndromes to acute myeloid leukemia

CHIP	MDS	AML
TP53	GATA2	CEBPA
DNMT3A	RUNX1	FLT3
TET2	EZH2	NRAS
ASXL1	STAG2	PTPN11
PPM1D	—	WT1
SRSF2	—	IDH1
—	—	IDH2

VAF greater than or equal to 10% is sufficient to be incorporated into the MDS/AML or AML categories. In contrast to the 3 distinct disease entities delineated under the ICC umbrella category, the WHO only designates MDS-bi*TP53* as a specific entity with blast percentage cutoff remaining at 0% to 19%.[1]

On the other hand, *NPM1* mutations, core binding factor rearrangements, and MLL/11q23 rearrangements are most commonly seen in de novo AML and very rarely in MDS or AML-MR.[29] Only 5.4% of secondary AML subjects carry *NPM1* mutations without concurrent *ASXL1*, *EZH2*, *BCOR*, *SF3B1*, *SRSF2*, *U2AF1*, *ZRSR2*, *STAG2*, or *TP53* mutations.[29] In addition, it has been shown that *NPM1* mutations in patients diagnosed with MDS with less than 20% blasts have better outcomes when treated with AML-based treatment approaches, such as intensive chemotherapy and stem cell transplantation, rather than MDS-based approaches, such as hypomethylating agents.[37] Studies for *KMT2A*, *MECOM*, and *NUP98* mutations have similarly demonstrated aggressive features at blast counts less than 20%; it is for these reasons that the WHO and ICC guidelines have lowered the blast threshold for these and other defining genetic abnormalities.[1,23,38–40]

Defining somatic mutations in the WHO and ICC guidelines include complex karyotype (≥3 abnormalities), 5q deletion or loss of 5q due to unbalanced translocation, monosomy 7, 7q deletion or loss of 7q due to unbalanced translocation, 11q deletion, 12p deletion or loss of 12p due to unbalanced translocation, 17p deletion or loss of 17p due to unbalanced translocation, isochromosome 17q, and idic(X) (q13).[1,2] The WHO guidelines also identify monosomy 13 or 13q deletion and the ICC guidelines identify trisomy 8 and 20q deletion as myelodysplasia-related somatic mutations.[1,2] The isolated deletion of 5q in particular is a common finding in patients with MDS and is associated with a more indolent subtype with anemia and thrombocytosis.[23,41]

CLINICAL THERAPIES

Historically, AML arising from MDS or with evidence of marked dysplasia was treated in a fashion similar to that used for de novo AML, with anthracycline-based chemotherapy regimens and strong consideration of allogeneic hematopoietic cell transplant as the only therapy with curative potential. With these approaches, retrospective reviews have repeatedly shown that outcomes in secondary AML are inferior to those seen with de novo AML, with lower rates of complete remission and frequent relapses.[42] Early efforts to improve treatment responses largely involved intensifying induction chemotherapy regimens, although these efforts were largely unsuccessful. Azacitidine (Aza) and decitabine are nucleoside analogues that incorporate into DNA and inhibit DNA methyltransferase. They have been extensively studied in MDS and secondary AML, given the importance of DNA methylation in progression from MDS to AML. The AZA-001 trial led to the approval of Aza for the treatment of MDS after showing a survival benefit compared with conventional care.[43] Of note, this study included patients with 21% to 30% blasts. An Aza-venetoclax combination has also been associated with complete response and complete remission with incomplete blood count recovery rate in AML with poor-risk cytogenetics and *TP53* mutations.[44] CPX-351, a liposomal encapsulation of cytarabine and daunorubicin, has been shown to be associated with significantly longer survival compared to conventional 7 + 3 in older adults with newly diagnosed secondary AML, with a safety profile similar to that of conventional 7 + 3 therapy.[45] With the creation of the MDS/AML group in the ICC classification, there will be a greater number of therapies available for patients with 10% to 19% blasts.

SUMMARY

In conclusion, advancements in the understanding of the genetic and molecular spectrum between MDS and AML have led to significant changes in the diagnostic criteria from the 2016 WHO guidelines to the current 2022 WHO and ICC guidelines. There is now a heavy emphasis on disease-defining genetic and molecular features and less emphasis on morphologic features and strict blast thresholds. With this shift away from blast percentages for diagnosis, there is more flexibility in the treatment options for patients with MDS and AML, as patients who did not meet the 20% blast cutoff and were classified as MDS under the 2016 WHO guidelines now have the opportunity to be reclassified as AML and qualify for more aggressive therapies. Preliminary studies assessing survival rates in patients previously diagnosed with MDS and reclassified under the 2022 WHO criteria have supported these changes.[46]

Although the diagnostic criteria for MDS and AML between the two classification systems are very similar, significant differences remain, particularly in the window between 10% to 19% blasts. The WHO guidelines remove the blast threshold for cases with defining genetic or molecular features but otherwise retain the 20% cutoff for cases without distinct abnormalities. The ICC guidelines set the blast threshold to 10% for cases with defining genetic or molecular features but also define cases between 10% to 19% blasts without distinct abnormalities under a new category, MDS/AML. Furthermore, some entities and mutations—such as *RUNX1*, monosomy 13 or 13q deletion, trisomy 8, and 20q deletion—are recognized by one classification system but not the other. These variations have important implications on future pathology reports, treatment strategies, and clinical trial inclusion criteria and will need to be recognized and appreciated moving forward.

CLINICS CARE POINTS

- Secondary AML represents a heterogenous group of patients with features often overlapping de novo cases with similar genetics.
- The historically poor outcomes in secondary AML reflect the higher proportion of negative features such as poor risk cytogenetics and *TP53* mutation.
- The latest editions of the WHO classification and the ICC further emphasize disease biology and genetic features while softening the boundary between MDS and AML.
- In both classifications, AML-myelodysplasia related, is defined by specific mutational or cytogenetic abnormalities and can no longer be defined by morphology alone.
- AML with mutated *TP53* is recognized as a new distinct entity in the ICC but not in the WHO and is defined by the presence of a pathogenic *TP53* mutation at a variant allelic frequency of greater than or equal to 10%.

DISCLOSURE

The authors have nothing to disclose.

REFERENCES

1. Khoury JD, Solary E, Abla O, et al. The 5th edition of the World Health Organization Classification of Haematolymphoid Tumours: Myeloid and Histiocytic/Dendritic Neoplasms. Leukemia 2022;36(7):1703–19.

2. Arber DA, Orazi A, Hasserjian RP, et al. International Consensus Classification of Myeloid Neoplasms and Acute Leukemias: integrating morphologic, clinical, and genomic data. Blood 2022;140(11):1200–28.

3. Ambinder AJ, DeZern AE. Navigating the contested borders between myelodysplastic syndrome and acute myeloid leukemia. Front Oncol 2022;12:1033534.

4. Greenberg PL, Tuechler H, Schanz J, et al. Revised international prognostic scoring system for myelodysplastic syndromes. Blood 2012;120(12):2454–65.

5. Greenberg P, Cox C, LeBeau MM, et al. International scoring system for evaluating prognosis in myelodysplastic syndromes. Blood 1997;89(6):2079–88.

6. Granfeldt Østgård LS, Medeiros BC, Sengeløv H, et al. Epidemiology and clinical significance of secondary and therapy-related acute myeloid leukemia: a national population-based cohort study. J Clin Oncol 2015;33(31):3641–9.

7. Borthakur G, Lin E, Jain N, et al. Survival is poorer in patients with secondary core-binding factor acute myelogenous leukemia compared with de novo core-binding factor leukemia. Cancer 2009;115(14):3217–21.

8. Bennett JM, Catovsky D, Daniel MT, et al. Proposals for the classification of the myelodysplastic syndromes. Br J Haematol 1982;51(2):189–99.

9. Bennett JM, Catovsky D, Daniel MT, et al. Proposals for the classification of the acute leukaemias. French-American-British (FAB) co-operative group. Br J Haematol 1976;33(4):451–8.

10. Harris NL, Jaffe ES, Diebold J, et al. The World Health organization classification of neoplastic diseases of the hematopoietic and lymphoid tissues. Report of the clinical advisory committee meeting, airlie house, Virginia, november, 1997. Ann Oncol 1999;10(12):1419–32.

11. Vardiman JW, Thiele J, Arber DA, et al. The 2008 revision of the World Health Organization (WHO) classification of myeloid neoplasms and acute leukemia: rationale and important changes. Blood 2009;114(5):937–51.

12. Vallespi T, Torrabadella M, Julia A, et al. Myelodysplastic syndromes: a study of 101 cases according to the FAB classification. Br J Haematol 1985;61(1):83–92.

13. Economopoulos T, Stathakis N, Foudoulakis A, et al. Myelodysplastic syndromes: analysis of 131 cases according to the FAB classification. Eur J Haematol 1987;38(4):338–44.

14. Mufti GJ, Stevens JR, Oscier DG, et al. Myelodysplastic syndromes: a scoring system with prognostic significance. Br J Haematol 1985;59(3):425–33.

15. Vardiman JW, Harris NL, Brunning RD. The World Health Organization (WHO) classification of the myeloid neoplasms. Blood 2002;100(7):2292–302.

16. Greenberg P, Anderson J, de Witte T, et al. Problematic WHO reclassification of myelodysplastic syndromes. Members of the international MDS study group. J Clin Oncol 2000;18(19):3447–52.

17. Arber DA, Orazi A, Hasserjian R, et al. The 2016 revision to the World Health Organization classification of myeloid neoplasms and acute leukemia. Blood 2016;127(20):2391–405.

18. Myelodysplastic syndromes (MDS) Recent Trends in SEER Age-Adjusted Incidence Rates, 2001-2019. Seer.cancer.gov. Available at: https://seer.cancer.gov/statistics-network/explorer/application.html?site=409&data_type=1&graph_type=2&compareBy=sex&chk_sex_1=1&chk_sex_3=3&chk_sex_2=2&hdn_rate_type=1&race=1&age_range=1&hdn_stage=101&advopt_precision=1&advopt_show_ci=on&hdn_view=0&advopt_show_apc=on&advopt_display=2#resultsRegion0. Accessed March 27, 2023.

19. Menssen AJ, Walter MJ. Genetics of progression from MDS to secondary leukemia. Blood 2020;136(1):50–60.

20. Hulegårdh E, Nilsson C, Lazarevic V, et al. Characterization and prognostic features of secondary acute myeloid leukemia in a population-based setting: a report from the Swedish acute leukemia registry. Am J Hematol 2015;90(3): 208–14.

21. Leone G, Mele L, Pulsoni A, et al. The incidence of secondary leukemias. Haematologica 1999;84(10):937–45.

22. Estey E, Hasserjian RP, Döhner H. Distinguishing AML from MDS: a fixed blast percentage may no longer be optimal. Blood 2022;139(3):323–32.

23. Zavras PD, Sinanidis I, Tsakiroglou P, et al. Understanding the continuum between high-risk myelodysplastic syndrome and acute myeloid leukemia. Int J Mol Sci 2023;24(5):5018.

24. Papaemmanuil E, Gerstung M, Bullinger L, et al. Genomic classification and prognosis in acute myeloid leukemia. N Engl J Med 2016;374(23):2209–21.

25. Haferlach T, Nagata Y, Grossmann V, et al. Landscape of genetic lesions in 944 patients with myelodysplastic syndromes. Leukemia 2014 Feb;28(2):241–7.

26. Papaemmanuil E, Cazzola M, Boultwood J, et al. Somatic SF3B1 mutation in myelodysplasia with ring sideroblasts. N Engl J Med 2011 Oct 13;365(15):1384–95.

27. Visconte V, Rogers HJ, Singh J, et al. SF3B1 haploinsufficiency leads to formation of ring sideroblasts in myelodysplastic syndromes. Blood 2012;120(16):3173–86.

28. Malcovati L, Karimi M, Papaemmanuil E, et al. SF3B1 mutation identifies a distinct subset of myelodysplastic syndrome with ring sideroblasts. Blood 2015;126(2): 233–41.

29. Lindsley RC, Mar BG, Mazzola E, et al. Acute myeloid leukemia ontogeny is defined by distinct somatic mutations. Blood 2015;125(9):1367–76.

30. Chen J, Kao YR, Sun D, et al. Myelodysplastic syndrome progression to acute myeloid leukemia at the stem cell level. Nat Med 2019;25(1):103–10.

31. da Silva-Coelho P, Kroeze LI, Yoshida K, et al. Clonal evolution in myelodysplastic syndromes. Nat Commun 2017;8:15099.

32. Walter MJ, Shen D, Ding L, et al. Clonal architecture of secondary acute myeloid leukemia. N Engl J Med 2012;366(12):1090–8.

33. Walter MJ, Shen D, Shao J, et al. Clonal diversity of recurrently mutated genes in myelodysplastic syndromes. Leukemia 2013;27(6):1275–82.

34. Makishima H, Yoshizato T, Yoshida K, et al. Dynamics of clonal evolution in myelodysplastic syndromes. Nat Genet 2017;49(2):204–12.

35. Sperling AS, Gibson CJ, Ebert BL. The genetics of myelodysplastic syndrome: from clonal haematopoiesis to secondary leukaemia. Nat Rev Cancer 2017; 17(1):5–19.

36. Zhang L, McGraw KL, Sallman DA, et al. The role of p53 in myelodysplastic syndromes and acute myeloid leukemia: molecular aspects and clinical implications. Leuk Lymphoma 2017;58(8):1777–90.

37. Montalban-Bravo G, Kanagal-Shamanna R, Sasaki K, et al. NPM1 mutations define a specific subgroup of MDS and MDS/MPN patients with favorable outcomes with intensive chemotherapy. Blood Adv 2019;3(6):922–33.

38. Issa GC, Zarka J, Sasaki K, et al. Predictors of outcomes in adults with acute myeloid leukemia and KMT2A rearrangements. Blood Cancer J 2021;11(9):162.

39. Fang H, Yabe M, Zhang X, et al. Myelodysplastic syndrome with t(6;9)(p22;q34.1)/DEK-NUP214 better classified as acute myeloid leukemia? A multicenter study of 107 cases. Mod Pathol 2021;34(6):1143–52.

40. Cui W, Sun J, Cotta CV, et al. Myelodysplastic syndrome with inv(3)(q21q26.2) or t(3;3)(q21;q26.2) has a high risk for progression to acute myeloid leukemia. Am J Clin Pathol 2011;136(2):282–8.

41. Giagounidis AA, Germing U, Aul C. Biological and prognostic significance of chromosome 5q deletions in myeloid malignancies. Clin Cancer Res 2006; 12(1):5–10.
42. Goasguen JE, Matsuo T, Cox C, et al. Evaluation of the dysmyelopoiesis in 336 patients with de novo acute myeloid leukemia: major importance of dysgranulopoiesis for remission and survival. Leukemia 1992;6(6):520–5.
43. Dombret H, Seymour JF, Butrym A, et al. International phase 3 study of azacitidine vs conventional care regimens in older patients with newly diagnosed AML with >30% blasts. Blood 2015;126(3):291–9.
44. Pollyea DA, Pratz KW, Wei AH, et al. Outcomes in patients with poor-risk cytogenetics with or without TP53 mutations treated with venetoclax and azacitidine. Clin Cancer Res 2022;28(24):5272–9.
45. Lancet JE, Uy GL, Cortes JE, et al. CPX-351 (cytarabine and daunorubicin) liposome for injection versus conventional cytarabine plus daunorubicin in older patients with newly diagnosed secondary acute myeloid leukemia. J Clin Oncol 2018;36(26):2684–92.
46. Zhang Y, Wu J, Qin T, et al. Comparison of the revised 4th (2016) and 5th (2022) editions of the World Health Organization classification of myelodysplastic neoplasms. Leukemia 2022;36(12):2875–82.

Transfusion Support of Patients with Myelodysplastic Syndromes

Juliana Guarente, MD[a],*, Christopher Tormey, MD[b]

KEYWORDS

- Myelodysplastic syndromes • MDS • Anemia • Thrombocytopenia • Transfusion
- Transfusion medicine • Alloimmunization

KEY POINTS

- In myelodysplastic syndromes (MDS), the most commonly affected cell line is the erythroid cells, and thus patients with MDS often require frequent red blood cell (RBC) transfusions.
- RBC transfusion may be used to improve functional capacity and quality of life in patients with MDS, while platelet transfusion is typically given prophylactically or acutely to prevent or treat bleeding.
- Despite the frequency of transfusion in patients with MDS, there are few well-defined guidelines for RBC and platelet transfusion support in this patient population.
- Transfusion of blood products is not without risk, both short-term and long-term, such as transfusion reactions and alloimmunization, and these risks need to be balanced with the benefits that transfusion may provide.
- Regular communication between clinicians and blood bank physicians is crucial to ensure that patients with MDS receive the most appropriate blood products.

INTRODUCTION

Myelodysplastic syndromes (MDS) are a heterogeneous group of hematopoietic disorders in which ineffective hematopoiesis results in dysplastic hematopoietic cells and peripheral cytopenias. Genetic mutations and chromosomal abnormalities underly the dyspoiesis, and the most commonly affected cell line is the erythroid cells. Almost 90% of patients with MDS are anemic at the time of presentation,[1] and in 80-85% of patients eventually diagnosed with MDS, symptoms of anemia are the presenting

a Department of Pathology and Genomic Medicine, Pathology Residency Program, Thomas Jefferson University Hospital, 111 South 11th Street Gibbon Building, Room 8220, Philadelphia, PA 19107, USA; b Department of Laboratory Medicine, Transfusion Medicine Fellowship, Yale University School of Medicine, Yale-New Haven Hospital, 55 Park Street, Floor 3, Room 329D, New Haven, CT 06511, USA
* Corresponding author. Juliana.Guarente@jefferson.edu

Clin Lab Med 43 (2023) 669–683
https://doi.org/10.1016/j.cll.2023.07.002
0272-2712/23/© 2023 Elsevier Inc. All rights reserved.
labmed.theclinics.com

complaint.[2] Almost 60% of patients are severely anemic on presentation, with hemoglobin <9 g/dL.[1]

As MDS is a malignant disease of myeloid stem cells, the only cure available is allogeneic hematopoietic stem cell transplant. Most patients with MDS do not meet eligibility criteria for a stem cell transplant, and thus they are treated to manage their disease, rather than cure it. Disease management in MDS can be divided into methods that attempt to modify the natural course of the disease itself, including chemotherapy, and methods that attempt to ameliorate the symptoms of the disease. It is in this area that patients with MDS rely heavily on supportive blood component transfusions.

As most patients are diagnosed with MDS in the latter decades of life,[3] and because older patients (as well as others) may have comorbid conditions that limit their tolerance of first-line therapies, many of these patients are managed (sometimes exclusively) with red blood cell (RBC) and platelet transfusions. In fact, about 50% of patients with MDS receive RBCs at some point during their disease course.[1] Despite the frequency of transfusion in patients with MDS, there are few well-defined guidelines for transfusion support in this patient population. Transfusion of blood products is not without risk, both short-term and long-term, and these risks need to be balanced with the clinical and quality of life benefits that transfusion may provide. As the majority of patients with MDS are stable enough to be managed as outpatients, this article will review the rationale behind RBC and platelet transfusion in outpatients with MDS, as well as potential adverse events associated with transfusion and relevant blood bank considerations.

Red Blood Cell Transfusion

Why should patients with myelodysplastic syndromes receive red blood cell transfusions?

In the absence of a curative treatment option for MDS, the goals of treatment typically fall into three categories: improve quality of life (QOL), prevent or manage complications associated with the disease, and slow progression of disease/improve survival. Improving survival or delaying disease progression is typically achieved with disease-modifying therapies, while RBC transfusions are considered supportive care and serve to improve QOL and potentially manage complications. Symptoms of anemia, such as headaches or palpitations can be uncomfortable, and can considerably impact a patient's QOL. Additionally, anemia can affect one's functional capacity–cognitive function, ambulation, and ability to perform activities of daily living–which will also impact QOL. Chronic anemia can also have significant effects on organ system function, most notably the cardiovascular system, and can lead to complications such as heart failure or myocardial infarction.

More than 85% of patients with MDS have chronic anemia that is refractory to treatment.[3] Anemia can be addressed at the source, by improving RBC production in the bone marrow, or can be compensated for, through transfusion. Unfortunately, augmenting RBC production in MDS often fails to be effective, may have intolerable side effects, and is expensive.[4] For example, fewer than 20% of patients may respond to erythropoietin,[5] and even when G-CSF is added, response may be less than 40%.[6] Additionally, certain agents used for MDS treatment may themselves be myelosuppressive, thus worsening a patient's baseline anemia. Thus, RBC transfusion is frequently the best, and is often the only, option for overcoming anemia as well as improving QOL for patients with MDS.[7]

Does red blood cell transfusion improve quality of life in patients with myelodysplastic syndromes?. Quality of life (QOL) is a multifactorial and predominantly subjective variable. QOL is even more difficult to study in a condition such as MDS, where diagnoses and subsequent symptoms are heterogeneous. Even patients with the same disease classification and prognostic category may have distinct assessments of their QOL.

Nonetheless, anemia is largely recognized as an important contributor to poor QOL in MDS. Symptoms of anemia, such as weakness and dyspnea, can be debilitating and significant, even when anemia is mild.[3] Therefore, treating anemia and improving oxygen-carrying capacity should theoretically lead to some improvement in QOL, though consensus is lacking. For instance, some publications examining the relationship between QOL and transfusion have shown improvements.[3,8] Challenging in the assessment of the available literature is that many studies assess QOL in patients with MDS who are transfusion-dependent versus those who are transfusion-independent. Such investigations have found that transfusion-dependence correlates with worse disease and thus patients likely have other factors contributing to poor QOL. Additionally, adhering to a rigorous transfusion regimen can be burdensome, which may lead to a net negative impact on QOL, even if the transfusions themselves provide symptomatic improvement.

Objective ways of assessing of QOL provide greater understanding of the therapeutic benefit transfusions may provide. In a 2019 study, St. Lezin and colleagues[9] investigated the effect of transfusion on QOL and functional status in 208 outpatients $\geq$50 years old with at least one benign or malignant hematology/oncology diagnosis. To assess QOL, fatigue- and dyspnea-related scores were measured, while functionality was assessed with distance traveled in a six-minute walk test. Patients were divided into two groups based on concurrent cancer treatment to avoid confounding, and were assessed before transfusion and five to ten days after transfusion. Transfusion was associated with a moderate improvement in fatigue scores, but there was no change in dyspnea scores. For all patients, distance in the six-minute walk test improved by a median of twenty meters, while for patients not on concurrent cancer treatment, distance improved by a median of thirty meters. It can often be difficult to interpret the effect of RBC transfusion on QOL results, as variables such as fatigue and dyspnea are subjective. Therefore, it is important to include parameters than can be more objectively measured and compared, such as exercise tolerance or cognitive tests, as we begin to further elucidate optimal transfusion guidelines in MDS.

Does red blood cell transfusion prevent complications in patients with myelodysplastic syndromes?. Anemia results in decreased oxygen-carrying capacity and poor organ perfusion. To compensate, the heart works harder, pumping more rapidly and with more force. Over time, this increased work can lead to the remodeling of heart muscle, particularly left ventricular hypertrophy, as well as tax the conduction system and the vasculature of the heart itself.

Although anemia affects all organ systems, cardiac effects are one of the most consequential complications of MDS, primarily due to the impact on comorbid cardiovascular disease in a typically older population.[10] A few studies have looked specifically at patients with MDS to determine the impact of anemia and transfusion on the cardiovascular system. In 2005, Oliva and colleagues[11] published a pilot study of thirty-nine patients to determine how chronic anemia in patients with MDS affected cardiac remodeling. Twelve transfusion-dependent and twenty-seven transfusion-independent patients underwent echocardiography, which showed cardiac remodeling in eleven of twelve versus thirteen of twenty-seven patients (p = 0.017). Hemoglobin level was also found to be an independent predictor of cardiac hypertrophy. Other studies have also shown increased coronary artery disease, myocardial infarction, and congestive heart failure in anemic patients with MDS.[12] The beneficial effects of transfusion on cardiac function need to be balanced with the negative impacts transfusions can have on the heart, namely conduction disorders and cardiomyopathy that result from iron overload, as will be discussed in a later section. Beyond the examination of cardiac disease prevention, few other studies have been published to examine the impact of improving anemia on other end-organ function and much work can be done in this area.

When should patients with myelodysplastic syndromes receive red blood cell transfusions?

There is not yet a consensus on the best scenario in which to provide RBC transfusion support to anemic patients with MDS. The AABB currently uses a specific hemoglobin threshold to recommend transfusion in hemodynamically stable inpatients, endorsing RBC transfusion in this patient population when hemoglobin falls below 7.0 g/dL.[13] This threshold was derived from the TRICC trial and others, based on endpoints chosen for critically ill inpatients in the intensive care unit.[14] As outpatients with MDS differ in many ways from the patients in the TRICC trial, it is often not appropriate to extrapolate this transfusion threshold to patients with MDS. The impact of restrictive transfusion on endpoints such as 30-day mortality are in most cases not pertinent to stable patients with MDS who are transfused as outpatients. A more liberal transfusion strategy may be required to achieve the endpoints most important to and relevant for patients with MDS.

In 2020, Stanworth and colleagues[15] published the results of a small feasibility study to examine the effects of restrictive versus liberal transfusion thresholds on QOL in patients with MDS. Thirty-eight patients from twelve sites in the UK, New Zealand, and Australia were randomized to restrictive (n = 20, 8.0 g/dL to maintain a hemoglobin of 8.5–10.0 g/dL) or liberal (n = 18, 10.5 g/dL, to maintain a hemoglobin of 11.0–12.5 g/dL) transfusion arms. The goal of the study was to demonstrate compliance with transfusion thresholds, and compliance was 86% in the intention-to-treat population, indicating that a future larger study of restrictive versus liberal transfusion in patients with MDS is likely feasible. Mean pre-transfusion hemoglobin for the restrictive arm was 8.0 g/dL, and was 9.7 g/dL for the liberal arm; 82 RBC units were transfused in the restrictive arm, while 192 RBC units were transfused in the liberal arm. Although this was a small study, an important outcome was shown–when compared to patients in the restrictive arm, patients in the liberal arm had improved QOL in the five main domains studied. This is may be reflective of the larger population of patients with MDS, as other studies have shown that many patients would often like to be transfused at higher hemoglobin thresholds.[16] The results of this feasibility study support the need for further studies of appropriate transfusion thresholds in patients with MDS.

An alternative to the strategy of establishing broad-based hemgloibin transfusion thresholds in MDS is to allow a patient's symptoms to guide when RBC transfusion may be indicated. In 2022, Vijenthira and colleagues[2] published the results of a survey of the experiences of 447 transfusion-dependent patients with MDS. In this study, a web-based survey was sent to patients with MDS in the US, Canada, and the UK; patients transfused within the previous 8 weeks were included. The survey included 57 questions pertaining to various aspects of transfusion, including questions regarding anemia-related symptoms, transfusion practice, and transfusion preferences, providing one of the most comprehensive pictures of the MDS patient transfusion experience to date.

One question asked in this study was "For how many days do you feel unwell (fatigue, short of breath, weak, and so forth) before receiving your next transfusion?"

64% of respondents reported feeling unwell for >5 days, while 2% of patients reported feeling unwell for <1 day. Respondents reported weakness and dizziness/lightheadedness, with fatigue and shortness of breath having the largest impact on their lives. Importantly, 8% of patients never reported feeling unwell prior to transfusion. Additionally, 26% of respondents expressed that higher hemoglobin thresholds for transfusion would improve their QOL. These differences stress the importance of a patient-guided approach to transfusion–the respondents who reported feeling unwell for >5 days were likely being under-transfused, while the respondents who never reported feeling unwell may have been over-transfused.

As was seen in these studies, patient input should be taken into account when determining ideal hemoglobin thresholds. Some countries have already begun incorporating patient-driven transfusion practices into their guidelines. For example, the British Committee for Standards in Haematology guidelines on the diagnosis and management of patients with MDS recommend that RBC transfusions be administered "to improve symptomatic anemia," rather than recommending a specific hemoglobin threshold.[17] Going forward, the transfusion community will need to find the optimal balance between patients' desire for more liberal transfusion practices and the negative effects of chronic RBC exposure.

What are the complications of red blood cell transfusion in myelodysplastic syndromes?

Although RBC transfusions can reduce complications of anemia and may improve QOL, the risks associated with RBC transfusion must always be considered. Side effects of transfusion can loosely be divided into sequelae that affect patients acutely or chronically. Acutely in the setting of a transfusion, patients may experience transfusion reactions, including febrile non-hemolytic transfusion reactions (FNHTR), transfusion-associated circulatory overload (TACO) or transfusion-related acute lung injury (TRALI). There is little data to suggest that patients with MDS are more (or less) vulnerable to these acute reactions than other chronically transfused populations. With chronic, repeated RBC transfusions patients are at risk of iron overload, as well as alloimmunization to RBC antigens, placing them at higher risk for delayed hemolytic transfusion reactions (DHTRs) with future transfusions. It is with these latter categories of chronic issues that MDS-specific concerns arise.

Red blood cell alloimmunization. When a patient is exposed to a blood group antigen he or she does not express on his/her own RBCs, an alloantibody may form against that antigen. Alloantibodies can then cause intravascular or extravascular hemolysis if the patient is again exposed to antigen-positive RBCs. Alloantibodies may fall below the limit of our ability to detect them using standard blood bank methods, called evanescence. However, alloantibody-producing plasma cells persist throughout life, and once a patient has developed an alloantibody, it must be "honored" for all future transfusions, meaning that all future transfusions must be negative for that antigen.

Not all patients who receive RBC transfusions are at risk of developing alloantibodies. In the general population, the rate of alloimmunization ranges from 1 to 10%.[18] Increased RBC exposure is associated with increased rates of alloimmunization. For example, patients with hemoglobin disorders such as thalassemia and sickle cell disease (SCD) are frequently transfused throughout life, and the rates of alloimmunization in these populations range up to 50% of transfused patients.[19–21]

As would be expected for a patient population that undergoes many RBC transfusions, patients with MDS also have increased rates of alloimmunization.[22] However, alloimmunization in patients with MDS is higher than other populations that are also frequently transfused, such as those with thalassemia or aplastic anemia. The reported incidence of alloimmunization in patients with MDS has ranged from 15 to 59%.[23–25] This higher rate of alloimmunization in patients with MDS was directly demonstrated in a 2015 retrospective study, where 56 patients with MDS were matched with 56 patients without MDS of the same age who had received the same number of RBC transfusions.[26] In patients with MDS, the alloimmunization rate was 27%, compared to 12% in patients without MDS.

It is interesting that overall, patients with MDS have higher rates of alloimmunization, especially in light of factors that tend to *decrease* antibody formation. Immunity generally wanes with aging, so for a disease with a median age of diagnosis in the mid-70s, it may be predicted that this patient population would have decreased alloimmunization. Additionally, studies have shown that patients being treated with hypomethylating agents such as azacitidine or decitabine have lower rates of alloimmunization than other patients with MDS.[27,28] What then can explain the overall increased rate of alloimmunization seen in patients with MDS? Studies have recently shown that an inflammatory microenvironment may play a key role in the pathogenesis of MDS,[29] and this inflammatory milieu may drive alloimmunization, as it does in SCD.[30]

Iron overload. Many patients with MDS have some degree of iron overload at baseline due to inefficient use of iron from ineffective erythropoiesis. Additionally, each unit of RBCs contains about 200–250 mg of iron. Most patients with MDS have no naturally occurring way of excreting iron (younger women will lose some iron with menstruation). Therefore, patients who undergo frequent RBC transfusions may begin to accumulate excess iron in various organs, such as the heart, liver, and pancreas. Iron accumulation in these organs can lead to cardiomyopathy, cardiac conduction problems, cirrhosis, and diabetes mellitus.

In other patient populations that are frequently transfused, including those with thalassemia and SCD, iron chelation has been shown to improve survival,[31] and is now the standard of care in these patients to reduce toxicity from iron overload. In a recent meta-analysis, Yang and colleagues[32] demonstrated that patients with MDS undergoing iron chelation therapy had a longer median overall survival. Multiple societies recommend iron chelation for patients with MDS, although there is not a consensus as to when chelation therapy should be initiated in this population.[17,33–35] Iron chelation therapies, such as deferasirox, deferiprone, and deferoxamine, can be difficult to tolerate, and though their benefit is evident, patients may not always be consistently compliant. A balance needs struck between frequent transfusion and iron chelation to prevent the negative effects of iron overload from overtaking the benefits of transfusion of QOL.

Transfusion reactions. Transfusion reactions, which are well-defined,[36] may be directly related to the transfusion of the indicated component (eg, hemolytic reactions secondary to transfusion of antigen-positive RBCs in an alloimmunized patient), related to other materials in the blood product (febrile reactions secondary to residual leukocytes), or related to how the component was transfused (volume overload secondary to rapid infusion). FNHTR is the most commonly reported acute transfusion reaction in patients with MDS, in line with what is seen in other populations.[37–39]

Although patients with MDS may experience all other types of transfusion reactions, TACO is particularly important to keep in mind in this population as patients with MDS are older and may have cardiovascular comorbidities at the time of diagnosis. Additionally, the iron overload resulting from numerous RBC transfusions over their disease course can lead to the development of cardiomyopathy and congestive heart failure.

Patients with MDS would generally benefit from slower transfusion, over a maximum of four hours. In patients especially at risk for volume overload, RBC units may be split in half, and each half unit may be transfused over four hours.

As discussed previously, patients with MDS are also at risk for DHTRs, due to the increased rate of alloimmunization and potential antibody evanescence in this patient population. If a patient presents to a new facility and needs a transfusion, and a prior antibody is not demonstrating, incompatible, antigen-positive RBCs may be inadvertently issued. With re-exposure to the antigen, an anamnestic response will ensue, alloantibody titers will increase, and the incompatible, antigen-positive RBCs will be attacked by the immune system. In most instances, the hemolysis will be slow and extravascular, and may go undetected because of the delayed onset, especially in outpatients. However, anti-Kidd antibodies are notorious for their tendency to evanesce rapidly, and can cause intravascular hemolysis (in one study anti-Jk^a antibodies were found in 21% of patients with MDS).[39] As such, it is important to obtain a full transfusion history for patients with MDS, including contacting blood banks at outside hospitals to determine if the patient has a history of any alloantibodies. Some have advocated for a national antibody registry in the United States, especially for patients with SCD[40]; this would be beneficial for the highly alloimmunized population of patients with MDS as well.

How should patients with myelodysplastic syndromes be transfused from a blood bank perspective?

All patients requiring RBC transfusion should have a type and screen performed to determine their ABO and Rh D type, and to assess for the presence of any alloantibodies to minor RBC antigens. If alloantibodies are found, RBCs negative for the corresponding antigen are provided. At present, there are no formal guidelines to match beyond ABO and Rh D for patients with MDS, although such approaches could potentially mitigate alloantibody formation (as is seen in SCD). More work in this area is needed and this topic is discussed at greater length later in this article.

Transfused RBCs (and platelets) should be leukoreduced to remove donor leukocytes. Most blood products transfused in the United States undergo pre-storage leukoreduction, which removes >99% of leukocytes and will decrease FNHTRs and CMV transmission. Leukoreduction also reduces HLA sensitization, which is important to decrease potential refractoriness for patients who may require multiple platelet transfusions, and for those who may go on to allogeneic HSCT.[41]

Do blood products for patients with myelodysplastic syndromes need to be irradiated?. Transfusion-associated graft versus host disease (TA-GVHD) is a nearly universally fatal, potential complication of transfusion.[42] In TA-GVHD, donor T-lymphocytes in cellular blood products (whole blood, RBCs, platelets, granulocytes) and liquid plasma attack recipient tissues, particularly skin and gastrointestinal epithelium, as well as bone marrow, which accounts for the lethality of TA-GVHD. Patients at risk for TA-GVHD are those who have a congenital immunodeficiency and those who are substantially immunosuppressed, as well as immunocompetent individuals who have a common HLA haplotype with the blood product donor.

Leukoreduction removes >99% of donor leukocytes; however, because TA-GVHD is almost invariably fatal, leukoreduction is not considered rigorous enough to eliminate GVHD risk.[42] Therefore, to fully prevent TA-GVHD, cellular blood products (as well as plasma that has never been frozen) must undergo gamma or X-ray irradiation before transfusion. Irradiation induces breakage of DNA, thus preventing the proliferation of any lymphocytes that may remain in the blood product.

As most patients with MDS are not candidates for allogeneic HSCT, they will never undergo the intense ablative chemotherapy or radiation that may put someone at risk for TA-GVHD. Therefore, most patients with MDS will not absolutely require irradiated RBCs. Chemotherapy regimens that may be used to treat MDS are not intense enough to cause a level of immunosuppression that would put someone at risk for TA-GVHD. However, if a patient is to undergo allogeneic HSCT, irradiated blood products should be provided beginning at the time conditioning chemotherapy or radiation are initiated.[42,43]

Should we provide antigen-matched red blood cells for transfusion in patients with myelodysplastic syndromes?. As discussed above, alloimmunization is prevalent in patients with MDS. Alloimmunization can make finding compatible RBCs difficult, may result in DHTRs, and can lead to difficulties during possible future stem cell transplantation.[44] In patients with SCD, alloimmunization is associated with decreased overall survival.[45] Some in the transfusion medicine community advocate for measures to prevent or reduce the formation of alloantibodies in patients with SCD, which could benefit patients with MDS as well.

Rh C/c and E/e, as well as K, are the most immunogenic RBC antigens after Rh D. Unsurprisingly, alloantibodies to these antigens are among the most commonly produced in patients with MDS.[23–25,28] To reduce alloimmunization, the antigen status of the patient can be determined, and antigen-matched blood products can then be provided. Antigen status can be determined either through phenotypic or genotypic methods. This may be performed for only the most immunogenic antigens (Rh C/c and E/e, as well as K, commonly referred to as "CEK matching") or may be extended to include other antigens such as Fy^a/Fy^b, Jk^a/Jk^b, and S/s. Ideally, antigen status would be determined at the time of MDS diagnosis, to prevent exposure to foreign RBC antigens during all future transfusions.

In patients with SCD, it has been shown that transfusion with RBCs matched for C/c, E/e, and K antigens can decrease rates of alloimmunization from 18-47% to 5-24%,[46] and multiple guidelines now recommend prophylactic matching for RBC antigens in the Rh (C/c, E/e) and Kell systems in patients with SCD.[47–49] In 2015, Guelsin and colleagues[50] found in a study of forty-three patients with MDS that alloantibody formation could be have been prevented in 68% of the patients if molecular matching had been performed for Rh C/c, E/e, and K. Additionally, in 2017 Lin and colleagues[51] performed a study of 176 transfusion-dependent patients with MDS and found that a policy of prophylactic antigen matching for Rh C/c, E/e, and K significantly reduced rates of Rh and Kell alloimmunization, but did not significantly reduce rates of alloimmunization overall. This is a population that would likely benefit from upfront testing and antigen matching for transfusions, especially extended matching, as patients with MDS have demonstrated that they are prone to develop new antibodies when challenged with foreign red blood cell antigens, even those that tend to be less immunogenic.

Few guidelines exist to guide the provision of antigen-matched RBC units for transfusion in patients with MDS. The British Committee for Standards in Haematology guidelines on the diagnosis and management of patients with MDS state that extended RBC phenotyping should be considered in patients who are regularly transfused, but does not specifically define what antigens should be matched, when in a patient's disease course this should be implemented, or define "regularly transfused."[17] In France, patients with MDS are transfused with Rh and Kell matched RBCs, a standard that must be implemented immediately after diagnosis. Interestingly, despite removing stimulation from the most immunogenic red blood cell antigens, alloimmunization remains high in this population (22.3% reported, most commonly to the Jk[a] antigen).[39] Additional prospective studies need to be done to determine the impact of antigen matching on alloimmunization in patients with MDS, and the most effective way to implement antigen matching for this patient population.

Platelet Transfusion

Although anemia is the predominant cytopenia in MDS, patients may have thrombocytopenia in addition to anemia (or rarely as the sole issue) – 40-65% of patients with MDS are thrombocytopenic and as many as 50% of patients may require platelet transfusion.[52] In addition to thrombocytopenia, MDS may also affect platelet function, with resultant decreased or defective aggregation.[53]

Why should patients with myelodysplastic syndromes receive platelet transfusions?
Severe thrombocytopenia (platelet count less than 20×10^9/L) occurs in about 17% of patients with MDS.[54] Thrombocytopenic patients have poorer prognosis and increased bleeding, which is ultimately the cause of death in 14-24% of patients with MDS.[54] Although data suggests that the risk for spontaneous bleeding only increases after the platelet count falls below about 6×10^9/L,[55] patients with MDS may be at risk for bleeding at higher platelet counts as their platelets may be dysfunctional. To prevent morbidity and mortality due to bleeding, platelet transfusions may be given prophylactically to sustain an adequate platelet count, or may be given therapeutically during active bleeding to augment hemostasis.

When should patients with myelodysplastic syndromes receive platelet transfusions?
Currently, there is no consensus as to when outpatients with MDS should be transfused. The 2015 AABB Clinical Practice Guideline on platelet transfusion recommends prophylactic platelet transfusion to reduce the risk of spontaneous bleeding for a platelet count of $<10 \times 10^9$/L specifically in inpatients.[55] The 2017 platelet transfusion guidelines published by the British Committee for Standards in Haematology specifically recommend that a "no prophylaxis strategy" be used for patients with MDS who are not receiving active treatment, based on the BCSH MDS guidelines published in 2014.[17,56] As discussed in the Red Blood Cell Transfusion section, it is difficult to extrapolate guidelines put in place for inpatients to the outpatient MDS population. Additionally, platelet transfusion thresholds may be even more difficult to establish than RBC transfusion thresholds in patients with MDS, as different patients may have varying levels of platelet dysfunction. Commonly adopted practice often sees platelet counts maintained at $>20 \times 10^9$/L in MDS outpatients, but this is an anecdotal practice in nature and not based on rigorous evidence.

What are the complications of platelet transfusion in myelodysplastic syndromes?
Alloimmunization. Platelets express ABO antigens on their surface, as well as Class I human leukocyte antigens (HLA) and human platelet antigens (HPA). They do not express Rh antigens (although whole blood-derived products may be 'contaminated' with RBCs expressing these antigens). Similar to RBC antigens, patients can develop alloantibodies to HLA and HPA after exposure during transfusion or pregnancy.

There is not a "hemolysis" equivalent in platelets, in the sense that platelet breakdown products are not harmful in the way RBC breakdown products are, thus it is not uncommon for 'ABO-incompatible' platelet transfusions to be provided. However, HLA antibodies can cause rapid destruction and clearance of incompatible platelets, rendering their therapeutic effect null, a process termed platelet transfusion refractoriness.

While platelet refractoriness is often attributed to immune/antibody-mediated causes, non-immune refractoriness is far more common, found in 80-90% of patients with poor platelet increments. Patients with MDS may demonstrate risk factors for non-immune refractoriness, including splenomegaly, DIC, fever, infection, and confounding medications.[52] If a cause of non-immune platelet refractoriness is identified, addressing that issue should improve the refractoriness. If no clear non-immune cause is identified and a patient with MDS continues to be platelet transfusion refractory, then investigation for immune/antibody-mediated refractoriness should ensue.

Immune/antibody-mediated refractoriness, accounts for about 9% of poor platelet incremenets in patients with MDS who receive regular platelet transfusions.[52] In this setting, and if significant numbers of HLA antibodies are found, compatible platelets can be provided, including crossmatched platelets (demonstrating no serological reactivity) or HLA-matched platelets may be provided and often yield superior platelet increments in comparison to random donor units.

Transfusion reactions. As with RBC transfusion, patients with MDS who receive platelet transfusions are at risk for transfusion-associated adverse events. Acute hemolytic transfusion reactions (AHTRs) are also a rare complication of minor incompatible platelet transfusions, as discussed later in discussion, wherein the *plasma* component of the platelet unit may contain ABO antibodies. The adverse events most important to keep in mind for patients undergoing platelet transfusions are TTI and allergic reactions.

Platelets are stored at room temperature with constant agitation for 5-7 days. Room temperature storage makes platelets a prime medium for pathogenic, particularly bacterial, growth. Multiple measures have been put in place to limit bacterial contamination, including culture and, most recently in the US, pathogen reduction technology, wherein psoralens in conjunction with UV light damage DNA leading to inhibited pathogen replication. Pathogen reduction results in significant pathogen destruction; however, it is not effective for all known pathogens and not available for all platelet transfusions. Therefore, vigilance for septic transfusion reactions is needed during platelet transfusion.

Platelet products can also contain a significant amount of donor-derived plasma. Consequently, platelet transfusions have a higher incidence of allergic reactions compared to RBC transfusion. Reactions may be minor, with only an urticarial rash/pruritus, or may be more severe, manifesting with anaphylaxis. Patients with repeated allergic transfusion reactions may benefit from premedication with antihistamines and, for severe reactions, potentially even corticosteroids. If patients continue to have breakthrough allergic reactions despite these measures, an alternative option is to use platelets stored in platelet additive solution (PAS), wherein 60-70% of the plasma is removed and replaced with a crystalloid solution. Such approaches have been shown to decrease allergic transfusion reactions.

How should patients with myelodysplastic syndromes be transfused from a blood bank perspective?

The short window of use makes a platelet inventory difficult to maintain and manage. Therefore, the ABO type is not of paramount importance when releasing platelets for transfusion. Minor incompatible platelets may contain anti-A, anti-B, and anti-A,B, in the plasma portion, which can theoretically cause hemolysis of recipient RBCs. Major incompatible platelets may have A or B antigens on their surface which are incompatible with the anti-A, anti-B or anti-A,B in the recipient's plasma. Both major and minor incompatible platelet transfusions are considered safe, however, it is important to remain watchful during out-of-group platelet transfusion, as minor mismatches with high-titer anti-A and anti-B can result in significant hemolysis.[57,58] While anti-A, anti-B or anti-A,B in the recipient's plasma could theoretically result in the premature destruction of major incompatible platelets, out of group platelet transfusions are still considered therapeutic. While anti-A, anti-B, and/or anti-A,B antibodies do not typically result in substantial platelet destruction, providing ABO-compatible platelets can be trialed in individuals demonstrating transfusion refractoriness.

Irradiation. As discussed in the Red Blood Cell Transfusion section, patients with MDS do not always require irradiated blood products. However, it is critical that HLA- or crossmatched platelets are irradiated. Pathogen reduction of platelets, now provided by many blood suppliers, obviates the need for irradiation due to DNA destruction.

SUMMARY

Even as additional treatment modalities are discovered and implemented for patients with MDS, transfusion will likely remain an integral aspect of supportive care for this patient population. We eagerly await future studies that will help to define a more evidence-based way to provide RBC and platelet transfusion support to patients with MDS. In the interim, transfusions will need to be optimized to balance the benefits of transfusion with the negative effects, such as iron overload and alloimmunization.

CLINICS CARE POINTS

- *PEARL*: In patients with MDS, a patient-guided approach to transfusion, as opposed to transfusion at a universal hemoglobin threshold, may be best.
- *PEARL*: Objective ways of assessing of QOL, such as cognitive tests or assessment of exercise tolerance, may provide greater understanding of the therapeutic benefit of RBC transfusions.
- *PITFALL*: Patients with MDS should only be transfused when absolutely necessary–it has been shown that patients with MDS have a higher rate of alloimmunization to RBC antigens, and thus they are at greater risk for hemolytic transfusion reactions.
- *PEARL*: This is a population that would likely benefit from upfront testing and antigen matching for transfusions, especially extended matching, as patients with MDS have demonstrated that they are prone to develop new antibodies when challenged with foreign red blood cell antigens, even those that tend to be less immunogenic.

DISCLOSURE

The authors have nothing to disclose.

REFERENCES

1. Malcovati L, Porta MGD, Pascutto C, et al. Prognostic factors and life expectancy in myelodysplastic syndromes classified according to WHO criteria: a basis for clinical decision making. J Clin Oncol 2005;23(30):7594–603.
2. Vijenthira A, Starkman R, Lin Y, et al. Multi-national survey of transfusion experiences and preferences of patients with myelodysplastic syndrome. Transfusion 2022;62(7):1355–64.

3. Ryblom H, Hast R, Hellström-Lindberg E, et al. Self-perception of symptoms of anemia and fatigue before and after blood transfusions in patients with myelodysplastic syndromes. Eur J Oncol Nurs 2015;19(2):99–106.

4. Cogle CR, Reddy SR, Chang E, et al. Early treatment initiation in lower-risk myelodysplastic syndromes produces an earlier and higher rate of transfusion independence. Leuk Res 2017;60:123–8.

5. Hellström-Lindberg E. Efficacy of erythropoietin in the myelodysplastic syndromes: a meta-analysis of 205 patients from 17 studies. Br J Haematol 1995; 89(1):67–71.

6. Hellström-Lindberg E, Ahlgren T, Beguin Y, et al. Treatment of anemia in myelodysplastic syndromes with granulocyte colony-stimulating factor plus erythropoietin: results from a randomized phase II study and long-term follow-up of 71 patients. Blood 1998;92(1):68–75.

7. Brechignac S, Hellstrom-Lindberg E, Bowen DT, et al. Quality of life and economic impact of red blood cell (RBC) transfusions on patients with myelodysplastic syndromes (MDS). Blood 2004;104(11):4716.

8. Nilsson-Ehle H, Birgegård G, Samuelsson J, et al. Quality of life, physical function and MRI T2* in elderly low-risk MDS patients treated to a haemoglobin level of $\geq$120 g/L with darbepoetin alfa $\pm$ filgrastim or erythrocyte transfusions. Eur J Haematol 2011;87(3):244–52.

9. Lezin E St, Karafin MS, Bruhn R, et al. Therapeutic impact of red blood cell transfusion on anemic outpatients: the RETRO study. Transfusion 2019;59(6):1934–43.

10. Oliva EN, Schey C, Hutchings AS. A review of anemia as a cardiovascular risk factor in patients with myelodysplastic syndromes. Am J Blood Res 2011;1(2): 160–6.

11. Oliva EN, Dimitrov BD, Benedetto F, et al. Hemoglobin level threshold for cardiac remodeling and quality of life in myelodysplastic syndrome. Leuk Res 2005; 29(10):1217–9.

12. Malcovati L, Porta MGD, Strupp C, et al. Impact of the degree of anemia on the outcome of patients with myelodysplastic syndrome and its integration into the WHO classification-based Prognostic Scoring System (WPSS). Haematologica 2011;96(10):1433–40.

13. Carson JL, Guyatt G, Heddle NM, et al. Clinical practice guidelines from the AABB: red blood cell transfusion thresholds and storage. JAMA 2016;316(19): 2025–35.

14. Hébert PC, Wells G, Blajchman MA, et al. A multicenter, randomized, controlled clinical trial of transfusion requirements in critical care. Transfusion Requirements in Critical Care Investigators, Canadian Critical Care Trials Group. N Engl J Med 1999;340(6):409–17.

15. Stanworth SJ, Killick S, McQuilten ZK, et al. Red cell transfusion in outpatients with myelodysplastic syndromes: a feasibility and exploratory randomised trial. Br J Haematol 2020;189(2):279–90.

16. Buckstein R, Starkman R, Lin Y, et al. Forty percent of MDs patients wish they received red blood cell transfusions at higher hemoglobin thresholds than they currently are: a multinational transfusion audit. Blood 2018;132(Supplement 1): 3092.

17. Killick SB, Carter C, Culligan D, et al. Guidelines for the diagnosis and management of adult myelodysplastic syndromes. Br J Haematol 2014;164(4):503–25.

18. Hendrickson JE, Tormey CA. Understanding red blood cell alloimmunization triggers. Hematology Am Soc Hematol Educ Program 2016;2016(1):446–51.

19. Fasano RM, Booth GS, Miles M, et al. Red blood cell alloimmunization is influenced by recipient inflammatory state at time of transfusion in patients with sickle cell disease. Br J Haematol 2015;168(2):291–300.
20. Ramsey G, Smietana SJ. Multiple or uncommon red cell alloantibodies in women: association with autoimmune disease. Transfusion 1995;35(7):582–6.
21. Papay P, Hackner K, Vogelsang H, et al. High risk of transfusion-induced alloimmunization of patients with inflammatory bowel disease. Am J Med 2012;125(7): 717.e1–8.
22. Hendrickson JE, Tormey CA. Red blood cell antibodies in hematology/oncology patients: interpretation of immunohematologic tests and clinical significance of detected antibodies. Hematol Oncol Clin North Am 2016;30(3):635–51.
23. Sanz C, Nomdedeu M, Belkaid M, et al. Red blood cell alloimmunization in transfused patients with myelodysplastic syndrome or chronic myelomonocytic leukemia. Transfusion 2013;53(4):710–5.
24. Stiegler G, Sperr W, Lorber C, et al. Red cell antibodies in frequently transfused patients with myelodysplastic syndrome. Ann Hematol 2001;80(6):330–3.
25. Novaretti MC, Sopelete CR, Velloso ER, et al. Immunohematological findings in myelodysplastic syndrome. Acta Haematol 2001;105(1):1–6.
26. Rozovski U, Ben-Tal O, Kirgner I, et al. Increased incidence of red blood cell alloantibodies in myelodysplastic syndrome. Isr Med Assoc J 2015;17(10):624–7.
27. Leisch M, Weiss L, Lindlbauer N, et al. Red blood cell alloimmunization in 184 patients with myeloid neoplasms treated with azacitidine - a retrospective single center experience. Leuk Res 2017;59:12–9.
28. Ortiz S, Orero MT, Javier K, et al. Impact of azacitidine on red blood cell alloimmunisation in myelodysplastic syndrome. Blood Transfus 2017;15(5):472–7.
29. Basiorka AA, McGraw KL, Eksioglu EA, et al. The NLRP3 inflammasome functions as a driver of the myelodysplastic syndrome phenotype. Blood 2016;128(25): 2960–75.
30. Guarente J, Hendrickson JE, Li F, et al. SRSF2 or TET2 mutations in patients with MDS predict increased red blood cell alloimmunization. Blood 2022; 140(Supplement 1):5706–7.
31. Ballas SK, Zeidan AM, Duong VH, et al. The effect of iron chelation therapy on overall survival in sickle cell disease and β-thalassemia: a systematic review. Am J Hematol 2018;93(7):943–52.
32. Yang S, Zhang MC, Leong R, et al. Iron chelation therapy in patients with low- to intermediate-risk myelodysplastic syndrome: a systematic review and meta-analysis. Br J Haematol 2022;197(1):e9–11.
33. National Comprehensive Cancer Network®. NCCN clinical practice guidelines in oncology (NCCN guidelines®). Myelodysplastic syndromes. Version 1.2018. Available at: https://www.nccn.org/professionals/physician_gls/pdf/mds.pdf. Accessed January 18, 2023.
34. Malcovati L, Hellström-Lindberg E, Bowen D, et al. Diagnosis and treatment of primary myelodysplastic syndromes in adults: recommendations from the European LeukemiaNet. Blood 2013;122(17):2943–64.
35. Fenaux P, Haase D, Sanz GF, et al. Myelodysplastic syndromes: ESMO clinical practice guidelines for diagnosis, treatment and follow-up. Ann Oncol 2014; 25(Suppl 3):iii57–69.
36. U.S. Centers for Disease Control and Prevention. The National Healthcare Safety Network (NHSN) Manual: Biovigilance Component v2.5. Atlanta, GA: Division of Healthcare Quality Promotion, National Center for Emerging and Zoonotic

Infectious Diseases. Available at: http://www.cdc.gov/nhsn/PDFs/Biovigilance/BV-HV-protocol-current.pdf. Accessed Jan 18, 2023.

37. Gupta P, LeRoy SC, Luikart SD, et al. Long-term blood product transfusion support for patients with myelodysplastic syndromes (MDS): cost analysis and complications. Leuk Res 1999;23(10):953–9.

38. Niscola P, Tendas A, Giovannini M, et al. Transfusions at home in patients with myelodysplastic syndromes. Leuk Res 2012;36(6):684–8.

39. Moncharmont P, Quittançon E, Barday G, et al. Adverse transfusion reactions in patients with aplastic anaemia or myelodysplastic syndromes. Vox Sang 2019; 114(4):349–54.

40. Williams LA, Lorenz RG, Tahir A, et al. High percentage of evanescent red cell antibodies in patients with sickle cell disease highlights need for a national antibody database. South Med J 2016;109(9):588–91.

41. Ratko TA, Cummings JP, Oberman HA, et al. Evidence-based recommendations for the use of WBC-reduced cellular blood components. Transfusion 2001;41(10): 1310–9.

42. Guidelines on gamma irradiation of blood components for the prevention of transfusion-associated graft-versus-host disease. BCSH Blood Transfusion Task Force. Transfus Med 1996;6(3):261–71.

43. Treleaven J, Gennery A, Marsh J, et al. Guidelines on the use of irradiated blood components prepared by the British Committee for Standards in Haematology blood transfusion task force. Br J Haematol 2011;152(1):35–51.

44. Balbuena-Merle R, Hendrickson JE. Red blood cell alloimmunization and delayed hemolytic transfusion reactions in patients with sickle cell disease. Transfus Clin Biol 2019;26(2):112–5.

45. Nickel RS, Hendrickson JE, Fasano RM, et al. Impact of red blood cell alloimmunization on sickle cell disease mortality: a case series. Transfusion 2016;56(1): 107–14.

46. Fasano RM, Sullivan HC, Bray RA, et al. Genotyping applications for transplantation and transfusion management: the emory experience. Arch Pathol Lab Med 2017;141(3):329–40.

47. Chou ST, Alsawas M, Fasano RM, et al. American Society of Hematology 2020 guidelines for sickle cell disease: transfusion support. Blood Adv 2020;4(2): 327–55.

48. Yawn BP, Buchanan GR, Afenyi-Annan AN, et al. Management of sickle cell disease: summary of the 2014 evidence-based report by expert panel members. JAMA 2014;312(10):1033–48.

49. Davis BA, Allard S, Qureshi A, et al. Guidelines on red cell transfusion in sickle cell disease. Part I: principles and laboratory aspects. Br J Haematol 2017; 176(2):179–91.

50. Guelsin GAS, Rodrigues C, Visentainer JEL, et al. Molecular matching for Rh and K reduces red blood cell alloimmunisation in patients with myelodysplastic syndrome. Blood Transfus 2015;13(1):53–8.

51. Lin Y, Saskin A, Wells RA, et al. Prophylactic RhCE and Kell antigen matching: impact on alloimmunization in transfusion-dependent patients with myelodysplastic syndromes. Vox Sang 2017;112(1):79–86.

52. Cheok KPL, Chhetri R, Wee LYA, et al. The burden of immune-mediated refractoriness to platelet transfusions in myelodysplastic syndromes. Transfusion 2020; 60(10):2192–8.

53. Girtovitis FI, Ntaios G, Papadopoulos A, et al. Defective platelet aggregation in myelodysplastic syndromes. Acta Haematol 2007;118(2):117–22.

54. Kantarjian H, Giles F, List A, et al. The incidence and impact of thrombocytopenia in myelodysplastic syndromes. Cancer 2007;109(9):1705–14.
55. Kaufman RM, Djulbegovic B, Gernsheimer T, et al. Platelet transfusion: a clinical practice guideline from the AABB. Ann Intern Med 2015;162(3):205–13.
56. Estcourt LJ, Birchall J, Allard S, et al. Guidelines for the use of platelet transfusions. Br J Haematol 2017;176(3):365–94.
57. Balbuena-Merle R, West FB, Tormey CA, et al. Fatal acute hemolytic transfusion reaction due to anti-B from a platelet apheresis unit stored in platelet additive solution. Transfusion 2019;59(6):1911–5.
58. Guarente J, Harach M, Gould J, et al. Dilution is not the solution: acute hemolytic transfusion reaction after ABO-incompatible pooled splatelet transfusion. Immunohematol 2019;35(3):91–4.

Treatment Considerations of Myelodysplastic Syndromes/ Neoplasms for Pathologists

Yazan F. Madanat, MD[a], Amer M. Zeidan, MBBS[b],*

KEYWORDS

• MDS treatment • Therapeutic scheme • Approach to MDS • Genomics in MDS

KEY POINTS

• Accurate management of myelodysplastic syndromes/neoplasms (MDS) relies heavily on having an accurate pathologic assessment, which in part relies on having a good bone marrow aspirate and biopsy specimen for evaluation.
• A complete pathologic evaluation must include cytogenetic analysis and next generation sequencing and in some cases fluorescent in situ hybridization panel for MDS.
• MDS-*SF3B1* and MDS with deletion 5q are the only two MDS subtypes with approved treatment options; luspatercept for MDS-*SF3B1* and lenalidomide for del(5q) MDS.
• Bone marrow cellularity is helpful in select cases to consider anti-thymocyte globulin + cyclosporine for the less common presentation of hypocellular/hypoplastic MDS.
• Hypomethylating agent therapy remains the gold standard for patients with higher-risk MDS. Allogeneic hematopoietic cell transplantation remains the sole potential curative option, for eligible patients.

GOALS

1. How the approach to a bone marrow report aids in MDS treatment decisions
2. Understand genomically defined MDS entities and the impact on management
3. Understand advantages and pitfalls of current prognostic scoring systems in MDS

INTRODUCTION

Myelodysplastic syndromes/neoplasms (MDS) are a group of heterogeneous clonal stem cell malignancies that lead to bone marrow failure and carry a risk of progression

[a] Eugene P. Frenkel M.D. Scholar in Clinical Medicine, Division of Hematology and Medical Oncology, Harold C. Simmons Comprehensive Cancer Center, UT Southwestern Medical Center, Dallas, TX, USA; [b] Section of Hematology, Department of Internal Medicine, Yale Cancer Center, Smilow Cancer Center, Yale University, New Haven, CT, USA
* Corresponding author.
E-mail address: amer.zeidan@yale.edu
Twitter: @MadanatYazan (Y.F.M.); @Dr_AmerZeidan (A.M.Z.)

Clin Lab Med 43 (2023) 685–698
https://doi.org/10.1016/j.cll.2023.07.003
0272-2712/23/© 2023 Elsevier Inc. All rights reserved.

to more advanced myeloid neoplasms, namely, acute myeloid leukemia (AML).[1,2] Outcomes for patients with MDS may be affected by race/ethnicity, exposure to prior chemotherapy/radiation therapy and age.[3–6] Additionally, disease characteristics including peripheral blood counts, bone marrow blast percent, chromosomal abnormalities and gene mutations which have been incorporated into prognostic scoring systems form the bases of outcome prediction for patients with MDS. The aforementioned disease characteristics are incorporated into the international prognostic scoring system (IPSS), its revised version (IPSS-R) and the molecular version (IPSS-M). IPSS-M is the most comprehensive and encompasses all aforementioned aspects of the disease.[7–9] The current treatment paradigm and grouping of patients into lower-risk MDS *vs* higher-risk MDS has heavily relied on the original IPSS where patients with low/intermediate-I risk scores are grouped together as lower-risk MDS and enrolled in lower-risk MDS clinical trials, and patients with intermediate-II/high risk scores are grouped together as having higher-risk MDS.[10,11] Most drugs that have received regulatory approval for the management of MDS relied on using the original IPSS as part of the inclusion criteria, and used the original FAB classification, which is listed in the drug labels.[12] The revised-IPSS was used in the Medalist clinical trial, which led to the approval of luspatercept for its use in patients with lower-risk MDS on April 3, 2020. The trial defined lower-risk MDS as having a very low/low or intermediate IPSS-R risk score.[13,14] In 2022, the molecular IPSS became available as an online risk calculator (IPSS-M Risk Calculator (mds-risk-model.com)). This will likely have a great impact on the design of future clinical trial and enrollment due to its higher accuracy for predicting leukemia-free and overall survival for patients with MDS. The key to approach MDS management and treatment options in a methodical way heavily relies on the quality of a bone marrow aspirate and core biopsy in addition to having an experienced hemato-pathologist given the rarity of this disease and nuances in defining morphologic dysplasia. In this review, we highlight major treatment decision points for the management of patients with MDS focusing on elements from a bone marrow biopsy report as the basis of our medical decision-making.

HOW PATHOLOGISTS AND CLINICIANS SHOULD COLLABORATE TO BETTER THERAPEUTIC DECISIONS IN MYELODYSPLASTIC SYNDROMES?
Establish Myelodysplastic Syndromes Diagnosis

The first and most essential element to treat a patient with MDS is establishing an accurate diagnosis. It is important to note that there are conditions that may mimic MDS and lead to morphologic dysplasia and/or macrocytic red blood cells or anemia. We recommend checking for folate deficiency, vitamin B12 deficiency, vitamin B6 deficiency (sideroblastic anemia), copper deficiency (which may be a result of excessive zinc intake) in addition to evaluation thyroid function tests as part of the initial evaluation to rule out MDS-like conditions. In addition, to inquire about specific medications (methotrexate, valproic acid, mycophenolate) and excessive alcohol intake which may also mimic MDS and should be added to the patients' medical history. Historically, patients with MDS required having cytopenias in at least one cell line, ≥10% dysplastic changes in one or more cell lineages in order to establish a diagnosis of MDS or have a defining cytogenetic abnormality, where a patient may have a diagnosis of MDS-unclassifiable (MDS-U).[15,16] In 2022, the fifth edition of the World Health Organization (WHO5) and the International Consensus Classification (ICC) published updates to MDS diagnosis and disease sub-classifications.[17,18] Per the WHO5 classification, morphologically driven entities including hypoplastic MDS and MDS with fibrosis were added, in addition to MDS with *SF3B1* (molecularly defined) and MDS with bi-allelic *TP53* inactivation and no longer focuses on the number of dysplastic cell lines. However, per ICC, a category of MDS/AML was introduced for patients with 10-19% blasts in the bone marrow [eliminating MDS with excess blast 2 category and dysplasia is not required], in addition to the molecularly defined entities of MDS-*SF3B1* [dysplasia not required] and MDS with mutated *TP53*. In addition, some mutations such as *NPM1* and *bZIP CEBPA* in the presence of ≥10% bone marrow blasts are now classified as AML (per ICC) and *NPM1* mutation positivity coins a diagnosis of AML irrespective of blast percent per WHO5 classification. Therefore, it is of utmost importance to wait on the final karyotype and full gene panel testing results to finalize and confirm a diagnosis of MDS. Some patients may initially be diagnosed as having clonal cytopenia of undetermined significance (CCUS) or lack evidence of a hematolymphoid malignancy based on the bone marrow morphology and flow cytometry results, and later establish a diagnosis of MDS based on cytogenetic and molecular findings, or may be initially diagnosed with MDS and then upstaged to AML based on having an *NPM1* mutation or an AML defining cytogenetic abnormality.[17,18] Given the complexity with establishing an accurate MDS diagnosis and new disease entities that are genomically defined, a discussion between hematopathologists and clinicians is of utmost benefit to incorporate the medical history, clinical presentation and impression with pathologic findings. Our institution issues a final comprehensive pathology report once the cytogenetic and mutation test results are obtained. This ensures there is a finalized report having the most accurate disease classification. Issuing a comprehensive finalized pathology report should ideally become a standard of care approach in MDS.

Step One–Bone Marrow Cellularity, Is it Relevant?

The first step when a clinical reads the final cellularity percent for age on a pathology report, one must look at the quality of the bone marrow aspirate and core biopsy as suboptimal samples often results in a lower bone marrow cellularity. In 2022, WHO5 classification, recognizes hypoplastic MDS (MDS-h) as its own entity due to potential to change management approach for those patients.[17] Hypoplastic MDS encompasses 10-15% of MDS patients where bone marrow cellularity is <30% and often times responds better to immunosuppressive therapy.[19,20] Horse anti-thymocyte globulin (ATG) plus cyclosporine may be the most widely used approach, however, the addition of eltrombopag improved responses for patients with aplastic anemia and has been incorporated into the national guidelines to consider triplet therapy for hypoplastic MDS.[21–23] In conclusion, horse ATG + cyclosporine ± eltrombopag should be considered in patients with hypocellular/hypoplastic MDS. The benefits of this treatment approach were noted to be most predictable in patients with <20% bone marrow cellularity (**Fig. 1**).

Step Two–How an Accurate Blast Percent Shapes Treatment Decision and Response

The original French American British (FAB) classification (1982) recognized that impact of blast on disease classification and risk. MDS was known as refractory anemia (RA) and patients with 5-20% blasts were classified as having refractory anemia with excess blasts (RAEB) delineating a higher risk entity.[24] Clinicians pay most attention to the bone aspirate morphology for blast % quantification in the bone marrow, however, flow cytometry establishes aberrancy in myeloid blasts and provides quantification, additionally, immunohistochemical stains may also be performed to confirm the blast percent, particularly if the aspirate smear is hemodilute or aparticulate or in cases that are associated with significant marrow fibrosis. Most patients with

Hematopathologic Approach to Myelodysplastic Syndromes

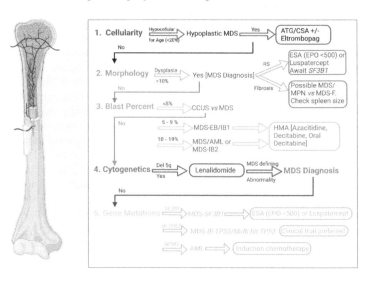

Fig. 1. How to incorporate bone marrow findings into MDSs treatment decisions. (Created with BioRender.com.) ATG, antithymocyte globulin; CSA, cyclosporine; ESA, erythropoiesis stimulating agents; MDS, myelodysplastic syndrome; MDS-f, MDS with fibrosis; MPN, myeloproliferative neoplasm; PO, erythropoietin.

lower-risk MDS have a blast percent of <5% in the bone marrow. MDS with excess blast (ICC) or MDS with increased blast-1 (MDS-IB1) per WHO5 may sometimes fall under a lower-risk MDS category per IPSS if the patient had normal cytogenetics and only 1 cytopenia per IPSS classification (hemoglobin <10 g/dL or absolute neutrophil count <1800/microL or platelet count <100,000/microL). This particular entity often poses a challenge for the management approach, particularly, when the cytopenia is not clinically significant (transfusion-independent anemia, mild-moderate thrombocytopenia without clinical bleeding, or mild-moderate neutropenia without having recurrent infections). While potentially controversial, for patients who are older and transplant ineligible, where the focus of therapy would be to improve blood counts and quality of life, patients with blasts of 5-6%, diploid cytogenetics and a single cytopenia (ie, IPSS Intermediate-1 risk) may be approached as having lower-risk MDS, where the management is guided based on mitigating the specific cytopenia, however, a clear discussion with those patients should be made and close monitoring with a repeat bone marrow biopsy considered to ensure stability of the blast percentage over time. The additional information from genomic panel testing and availability of IPSS-M would help further inform treatment decisions and consideration to approach such a patient as having a higher-risk MDS. Patients who are younger or transplant eligible, where the ultimate goal is curative, may be considered for a higher-risk MDS treatment approach. Patients with 10-19% bone marrow blasts, classified as MDS/AML per ICC and MDS-IB2 per WHO5 often times have higher-risk MDS and proceed with hypomethylating agent therapy (azacitidine, Decitabine, or decitabine-cedazuridine). Importantly, for treatment response assessment, accurate blast % quantification is key, as patients with $\leq$5% have a bone marrow CR when accompanied with a 50% reduction in blast percent from baseline. Per IPSS, blast categories include <5%, 5-10%, 11-20%, and 21-30%, however, per revised-IPSS, blast categories include $\leq$2%, >2% to <5%, 5-10%, >10%.[7,8] Per the IPSS and revised IPSS (which is the basis for molecular IPSS), patients with blasts of 5-10% have similar points added to the scoring system i.e. similar MDS risk, however, per current and previous WHO classifications, blasts of 10% would be classified as having a higher-risk disease category (MDS/AML per ICC or MDS-IB2 per WHO5). Additionally, current MDS response criteria indicate a blast percent of 5% or less is adequate to achieve a marrow complete remission.[25] It would be useful to consider unifying the disease classification, response criteria blast percent to align with the current prognostic scoring systems in the future. A proposed approach may be to consider revising a bone marrow CR response using a blast threshold of <5% [in line with AML response criteria], a single disease classification for blasts between 5 and 10% to align with IPSS/revised-IPSS and a single disease risk/classification for patients with >10% blasts for MDS/AML or MDS-IB2 to align with revised IPSS risk categories.

Step Three–Cytogenetics and Impact on Diagnosis, Risk, and Treatment Considerations

The impact of cytogenetics on establishing a diagnosis of MDS has changed over time.[12,26,27] In 2008, MDS-unclassifiable was specifically introduced when the clinical and laboratory features are consistent with MDS, however, the morphology is inconclusive, the following cytogenetic abnormalities made a presumptive diagnosis of MDS possible (MDS-U).[15] These included, unbalanced abnormalities monosomy 5, monosomy 7, monosomy 13, del(7q), del(5q), i(17q) or t(17p), del(13q), del(11q) del(12p) or t(12p), del(9q) or idic(X) (q13). In addition to the following balanced cytogenetic abnormalities, t(11;16), t(3;21), t(1;3), t(2;11), inv(3) and t(6;9). Additionally, complex karyotype defined as having three or more cytogenetic abnormalities was also MDS defining. These same cytogenetic abnormalities remained MDS defining in a cytopenic patient in the absence of dysplasia and were classified as MDS-U in 2016.[16] Important to note, deletion Y, trisomy 8 or deletion 20q were not considered to be MDS-defining in the absence of morphologic dysplasia. In 2022, the WHO5 classification removed MDS-U as a disease classification, and per ICC– only monosomy 7, deletion 7q, or complex karyotype were MDS defining and a diagnosis of MDS-not otherwise specified (MDS-NOS) can be made in the presence of the aforementioned chromosomal abnormalities.[17,28] We suspect this may lead to a substantial increase in the number of patients diagnosed with clonal cytopenia of undetermined significance (CCUS) for those patients previously diagnosed as MDS-U, and given that those patients are therapeutically approached as having lower-risk MDS, they would not be eligible to enroll in clinical trials for lower-risk MDS moving forward.

Chromosomal analysis results not only affect establishing an MDS diagnosis, but aid in risk stratification and impact prognosis in MDS. This has been recognized in the original IPSS where three cytogenetic risk groups were identified. Good risk cytogenetics included diploid karyotype, deletion Y, del(5q) and del(20q). Poor risk included complex ($\geq$3 abnormalities) and chromosome 7 abnormalities, whereas intermediate risk included all others. This was further subdivided into five risk groups in the revised IPSS. Very good risk included −Y, del(11q). Good risk included Normal, del(5q), del(12p), del(20q) and double including del(5q). Intermediate risk: del(7q), +8, +19, i(17q), any other single, double not including del(5q) or −7/del(7q), or independent clones. Poor risk cytogenetics: −7, inv(3)/t(3q)/del(3q), double including −7/del(7q), complex (3 abnormalities). Very poor risk included complex karyotype with >3 abnormalities. The latter on its own (4.0 points per R-IPSS) places a patient's MDS in a higher-risk MDS group.[23]

Lastly, cytogenetics impact MDS disease classification, where MDS with deletion 5q, first described in 1974,[29] remains its own disease entity since 2001 WHO classification[30] and has led to therapeutic advances. Lenalidomide received regulatory approval for the management of MDS with deletion 5q for patients with transfusion-dependent anemia and lower-risk disease per IPSS (low or intermediate-1 risk). Of 148 patients enrolled, transfusion independence rate was 67% with a median time to transfusion independence of 4.6 weeks. Of note, complete cytogenetic responses were seen in 45% of patients.[10,31–34] (see **Fig. 1**, **Table 1**).

Step Four–How Do Gene Mutations Impact Management

Molecular abnormalities are now widely recognized to play a major role in MDS pathogenesis, affecting disease risk and outcomes for patients with MDS.[35–37] Molecular characterization of MDS has been described in a few large patient cohorts.[38,39] In 2022, molecular abnormalities have been incorporated in the molecular-IPSS scoring system, which builds on the revised IPSS using this online calculator (IPSS-M Risk Calculator (mds-risk-model.com)).[9] Real world validation of the molecular IPSS demonstrated superiority over the revised IPSS for predicting leukemia free- and overall survival. The group validated their findings in patients without molecular testing, for predicting disease relapse and post-transplant survival. However, IPSS-M failed to predict response to hypomethylating agents; response duration and overall survival were inversely related to IPSS-M risk score.[40] Although molecular abnormalities' impact on response in MDS has been described, to date, no single/mutational combination should prevent a patient with higher-risk disease from receiving hypomethylating agent therapy.[41] (see **Table 1**).

Two molecular abnormalities currently influence MDS disease classification and aid in making a diagnosis of MDS; those include *SF3B1* and *TP53* mutations. Mutations in *SF3B1* have been investigated in several studies, portend favorable outcomes, and are frequently associated with ring-sideroblasts.[42–45] *TP53* mutations on the other hand, portend poor outcomes, particularly when there are two *TP53* mutations (ie, multi-hit) or bi-allelic in-activation where one mutation is associated with deletion 17p or copy neutral loss of heterozygosity (cnLOH) or monosomy 17.[3,46–49] Per ICC, a diagnosis of MDS-*SF3B1* can be made with having an *SF3B1* at a variant allele frequency (VAF) of ≥10%, and MDS with mutated *TP53* defined by having 2 distinct TP53 mutations (each VAF > 10%) or a single TP53 mutation with del(17p) or VAF >50% or cnLOH at 17p TP53 locus.[18] Minor differences exist per WHO5 classification where a genetically defined MDS entity includes: MDS-*SF3B1* (no VAF mandate), additionally, MDS with bi-allelic *TP53* (MDS-bi*TP53*) defined as having two or more *TP53* mutations or one mutation with evidence of *TP53* cnLOH.[17]

Molecular abnormalities in MDS aid in treatment decisions when it comes to MDS-*SF3B1*, where luspatercept, a recombinant fusion protein that binds transforming growth factor β superfamily ligands to reduce SMAD2 and SMAD3 signaling has received regulatory approval for patients with lower-risk MDS (revised-IPSS very low, low or intermediate risk), who are red blood cell transfusion dependent. Thirty eight percent of patients achieved the primary end-point of 8-week transfusion independence. Long-term benefits of luspatercept continued to be seen with possible improvement in neutrophil and platelet counts.[13,14,50–52] (see **Fig. 1**)

Table 1
Food and drug administration (FDA) approved therapies in MDS

FDA Approved	MOA/Drug Class	IPSS Risk (Inclusion Criteria)	Response Rate (%)	Overall Survival (Months)	Reference
Lenalidomide [MDS-del(5q)]	Immunomodulatory effects and Ubiquitination of CK1a and IKZF1	Low/Intermediate 1	8-week transfusion independence 67%	NA	List et al,[33] 2006
Luspatercept [MDS-SF3B1]	TGF-β ligand trap	Low/Intermediate 1	8-week transfusion independence 37.9%	NA	Fenaux et al,[13] 2020
Azacitidine	Hypomethylating agents	Intermediate-2 or high risk	CR 17% PR 12% HI-E 40%	24.5 mo vs 15 mo (PL)	Fenaux et al,[65] 2009
Decitabine		Intermediate-1/2 or high risk	CR 9% PR 8% HI 13%	14 mo vs 14.9 mo (PL)	Kantarjian et al,[66] 2006
Decitabine-cedazuridine		Intermediate-1/2 or high risk	CR 21% PR 0 mCR + HI 7% HI 16%	18.3 mo	Garcia-Manero et al,[67] 2020
Off-label Use					
Epoetin alpha Darbepoetin	Erythropoiesis stimulating agent	Low/Intermediate-1 Low/Intermediate 1	ER 31.8% vs 4.4% PL ER 38-72%	NA NA	Fenaux et al,[68] 2018 Park et al,[69] 2016
Lenalidomide in non-del(5q)	Immunomodulatory effects and Ubiquitination of CK1a and IKZF1	Low/Intermediate 1	8-week TI 26.9%	NA	Santini et al,[70] 2016
Lower-dose HMA (Azacitidine or Dectabine)	Hypomethylating agents	Low/Intermediate 1	CR 37% mCR 7% HI 18%	NA	Jabbour et al,[71] 2017

(continued on next page)

Table 1
(continued)

FDA Approved	MOA/Drug Class	IPSS Risk (Inclusion Criteria)	Response Rate (%)	Overall Survival (Months)	Reference
Horse-ATG plus cyclosporine	Immunosuppressive therapy	Low/Intermediate 1	ORR 48.8% CR 11.2% TI 30%	47.7 mo	Stahl et al,[21] 2018
Ivosidenib	IDH1 inhibitor	Higher-risk, R/R	ORR 81% CR 44%	NA	Sallman et al,[57] 2022
Enasidenib	IDH2 inhibitor	Higher-risk, R/R	ORR 35% CR 22%	20 mo	DiNardo et al,[59] 2022
Olutasidenib	IDH1 inhibitor	Higher-risk	ORR 33% CR 17% n = 6	NA	Watts et al,[60] 2023

Mechanisms of primary resistance to luspatercept are less clear and whether SF3B1 hotspot mutations impact response to therapy will need to be further investigated.[53] Spliceosome inhibitors that have gone through clinical trials have not shown great response despite on target effects.[54,55] Although *IDH1* and *IDH2* mutations are rare in MDS, they should be tested for as there are targeted therapy options including enasidenib [*IDH2* inhibitor], ivosidenib [*IDH1* inhibitor] and olutasidenib [*IDH1* inhibitor] approved in acute myeloid leukemia and have been investigated in patients with MDS.[56–61]

SUMMARY

Clinicians heavily rely on collaborating with our hematopathology teams to reach a reliable MDS diagnosis. Better understanding MDS biology and pathophysiology has led to the incorporation of molecular abnormalities in the disease risk stratification (IPSS-M) or disease classification (MDS-*SF3B1* or MDS-*TP53*). The blast percent cut offs, particularly 5-10% remain a single group per IPSS/revised IPSS, however, may have different disease classification per WHO5/ICC particularly for patients with 10% blasts. MDS response criteria often times rely on blast count enumeration in addition to laboratory criteria, therefore, a reliable bone marrow aspirate sample is key to assess treatment response. The treatment for lower-risk MDS continues to rely on improving blood counts, transfusion independence and improving quality of life, whereas, treatment for higher-risk MDS is aimed at delaying progression to AML and improving overall survival. A discussion between hematopathologists and clinicians is key to establish the most accurate MDS disease classification.

FUTURE DIRECTIONS

Unifying the WHO5 and ICC classification[62] as soon as possible will be important. Efforts for a combined classification have begun through different avenues including a data-drive initiative through the international consortium for MDS. The consortium has implemented efforts to re-evaluate and revamp response criteria for lower and higher-risk MDS. Incorporation of VAF will likely be necessary as a standard when reporting mutation test results using various next-generation sequencing panels to improve disease classification and risk stratification. Patients with suboptimal bone marrow biopsies may now be falsely classified as CCUS, therefore, clearly indicating the need for a repeat a bone marrow biopsy will be important by pathologists given the lack of "MDS-unclassifiable" entity in the new classification. Over the next decade and with advances in machine learning algorithms, we envision the ability to incorporate image recognition patterns through machine learning algorithms to help establish an MDS diagnosis and artificial intelligence to standardize the detection of quantification of morphologic dysplasia which may reduce inter-observer variability.[63] We also envision the ability to perhaps make a diagnosis of MDS without the need for a bone marrow biopsy as our understanding of the outcomes and disease course for patients with CCUS improves with time. A recent study presented at the annual society of hematology meeting devised a new classification of MDS irrespective of bone marrow blast counts.[64] Ultimately, we hope to be able to base our disease classification and clinical decision making more using clinical characteristics and disease biology. Mutational variant allele frequency has not been widely studied and incorporating VAF to help better understand driver and secondary hit mutations, and how those may influence choice of therapy and response to therapy will likely be better delineated in future studies. Treatments that alter the disease biology and natural history of the disease will be key to improve MDS patient outcomes.

CLINICS CARE POINTS

- Working closely with hematopathologisits is key to ensure patients with MDS are accurately diagnosed.
- Patients with lower-risk MDS have a few FDA approved options including lenalidomide, luspatercept and HMA therapy.
- Patients with higher-risk MDS only have HMA therapy as an approved option, but may have targeted therapy options approved in the near future.

DISCLOSURE

Y.F. Madanat has received honoraria/consulting fees from BluePrint Medicines, GERON, OncLive, and MD Education. Y.F. Madanat participated in advisory boards and received honoraria from Sierra Oncology, Stemline Therapeutics, Blueprint Medicines, Morphosys, Taiho Oncology, Rigel Pharmaceuticals, and Novartis. Y.F. Madanat received travel reimbursement from Blueprint Medicines and Morphosys. A.M. Zeidan received research funding (institutional) from Celgene/BMS, United States, Abbvie, United States, Astex, United States, Pfizer, United States, MedImmune/Astra-Zeneca, United Kingdom, Boehringer Ingelheim, United States, Trovagene/Cardiff oncology, Incyte, United States, Takeda, United States, Novartis, Switzerland, Aprea, and ADC Therapeutics; participated in advisory boards and/or had a consultancy with and received honoraria from AbbVie, Otsuka, Pfizer, Celgene/BMS, Jazz, Incyte, Agios, Boehringer-Ingelheim, Novartis, Acceleron, Astellas, Daiichi Sankyo, Cardinal Health, Taiho, Seattle Genetics, BeyondSpring, Cardiff Oncology, Takeda, Ionis, Amgen, Janssen, Epizyme, Syndax, Gilead, Kura, Chiesi, ALX Oncology, BioCryst, and Tyme; served on clinical trial committees for Novartis, Abbvie, Geron, and Celgene/BMS. *None of these relationships were related to this work. Figures are created with Biorender.com.*

REFERENCES

1. Rollison DE, Howlader N, Smith MT, et al. Epidemiology of myelodysplastic syndromes and chronic myeloproliferative disorders in the United States, 2001-2004, using data from the NAACCR and SEER programs. Blood 2008;112(1):45–52.
2. Zeidan AM, Shallis RM, Wang R, et al. Epidemiology of myelodysplastic syndromes: why characterizing the beast is a prerequisite to taming it. Blood Rev 2019;34:1–15.
3. Weinberg OK, Siddon A, Madanat YF, et al. TP53 mutation defines a unique subgroup within complex karyotype de novo and therapy-related MDS/AML. Blood Adv 2022;6(9):2847–53.
4. Goksu SY, Ozer M, Goksu BB, et al. The impact of race and ethnicity on outcomes of patients with myelodysplastic syndromes: a population-based analysis. Leuk Lymphoma 2022;63(7):1651–9.
5. Abou Zahr A, Kavi AM, Mukherjee S, et al. Therapy-related myelodysplastic syndromes, or are they? Blood Rev 2017;31(3):119–28.
6. Kuendgen A, Nomdedeu M, Tuechler H, et al. Therapy-related myelodysplastic syndromes deserve specific diagnostic sub-classification and risk-stratification-an approach to classification of patients with t-MDS. Leukemia 2021;35(3):835–49.

7. Greenberg P, Cox C, LeBeau MM, et al. International scoring system for evaluating prognosis in myelodysplastic syndromes. Blood 1997;89(6):2079–88.

8. Greenberg PL, Tuechler H, Schanz J, et al. Revised international prognostic scoring system for myelodysplastic syndromes. Blood 2012;120(12):2454–65.

9. Bernard E, Tuechler H, Greenberg PL, et al. Molecular international prognostic scoring system for myelodysplastic syndromes. NEJM Evidence 2022;1(7). EVIDoa2200008.

10. Fenaux P, Ades L. How we treat lower-risk myelodysplastic syndromes. Blood 2013;121(21):4280–6.

11. Sekeres MA, Cutler C. How we treat higher-risk myelodysplastic syndromes. Blood 2014;123(6):829–36.

12. Nosslinger T, Reisner R, Koller E, et al. Myelodysplastic syndromes, from French-American-British to World Health Organization: comparison of classifications on 431 unselected patients from a single institution. Blood 2001;98(10):2935–41.

13. Fenaux P, Platzbecker U, Mufti GJ, et al. Luspatercept in patients with lower-risk myelodysplastic syndromes. N Engl J Med 2020;382(2):140–51.

14. Garcia-Manero G, Mufti GJ, Fenaux P, et al. Neutrophil and platelet increases with luspatercept in lower-risk MDS: secondary endpoints from the MEDALIST trial. Blood 2022;139(4):624–9.

15. Vardiman JW, Thiele J, Arber DA, et al. The 2008 revision of the World Health Organization (WHO) classification of myeloid neoplasms and acute leukemia: rationale and important changes. Blood 2009;114(5):937–51.

16. Arber DA, Orazi A, Hasserjian R, et al. The 2016 revision to the World Health Organization classification of myeloid neoplasms and acute leukemia. Blood 2016; 127(20):2391–405.

17. Khoury JD, Solary E, Abla O, et al. The 5th edition of the world Health organization classification of haematolymphoid tumours: myeloid and histiocytic/dendritic neoplasms. Leukemia 2022;36(7):1703–19.

18. Arber DA, Orazi A, Hasserjian RP, et al. International consensus classification of myeloid neoplasms and acute leukemias: integrating morphologic, clinical, and genomic data. Blood 2022;140(11):1200–28.

19. Bennett JM, Orazi A. Diagnostic criteria to distinguish hypocellular acute myeloid leukemia from hypocellular myelodysplastic syndromes and aplastic anemia: recommendations for a standardized approach. Haematologica 2009;94(2): 264–8.

20. Locatelli F, Strahm B. How I treat myelodysplastic syndromes of childhood. Blood 2018;131(13):1406–14.

21. Stahl M, DeVeaux M, de Witte T, et al. The use of immunosuppressive therapy in MDS: clinical outcomes and their predictors in a large international patient cohort. Blood Adv 2018;2(14):1765–72.

22. Peffault de Latour R, Kulasekararaj A, Iacobelli S, et al. Eltrombopag added to immunosuppression in severe aplastic anemia. N Engl J Med 2022;386(1):11–23.

23. Greenberg PL, Stone RM, Al-Kali A, et al. NCCN guidelines(R) insights: myelodysplastic syndromes, version 3.2022. J Natl Compr Cancer Netw 2022;20(2): 106–17.

24. Bennett JM, Catovsky D, Daniel MT, et al. Proposals for the classification of the myelodysplastic syndromes. Br J Haematol 1982;51(2):189–99.

25. Cheson BD, Greenberg PL, Bennett JM, et al. Clinical application and proposal for modification of the International Working Group (IWG) response criteria in myelodysplasia. Blood 2006;108(2):419–25.

26. West RR, Stafford DA, White AD, et al. Cytogenetic abnormalities in the myelo-dysplastic syndromes and occupational or environmental exposure. Blood 2000;95(6):2093–7.

27. Schanz J, Tuchler H, Sole F, et al. New comprehensive cytogenetic scoring system for primary myelodysplastic syndromes (MDS) and oligoblastic acute myeloid leukemia after MDS derived from an international database merge. J Clin Oncol 2012;30(8):820–9.

28. Adema V, Ma F, Kanagal-Shamanna R, et al. Targeting the EIF2AK1 signaling pathway rescues red blood cell production in SF3B1-mutant myelodysplastic syndromes with ringed sideroblasts. Blood Cancer Discov 2022;3(6):554–67.

29. Van den Berghe H, Cassiman JJ, David G, et al. Distinct haematological disorder with deletion of long arm of no. 5 chromosome. Nature 1974;251(5474):437–8.

30. Vardiman JW, Harris NL, Brunning RD. The World Health Organization (WHO) classification of the myeloid neoplasms. Blood 2002;100(7):2292–302.

31. Chng WJ. Treatment of myelodysplastic syndromes. N Engl J Med 2005;352(20): 2134–5 [author reply: 2134-2135].

32. List A, Kurtin S, Roe DJ, et al. Efficacy of lenalidomide in myelodysplastic syndromes. N Engl J Med 2005;352(6):549–57.

33. List A, Dewald G, Bennett J, et al. Lenalidomide in the myelodysplastic syndrome with chromosome 5q deletion. N Engl J Med 2006;355(14):1456–65.

34. Raza A, Reeves JA, Feldman EJ, et al. Phase 2 study of lenalidomide in transfusion-dependent, low-risk, and intermediate-1 risk myelodysplastic syndromes with karyotypes other than deletion 5q. Blood 2008;111(1):86–93.

35. Bejar R, Levine R, Ebert BL. Unraveling the molecular pathophysiology of myelo-dysplastic syndromes. J Clin Oncol 2011;29(5):504–15.

36. Bejar R, Stevenson KE, Caughey BA, et al. Validation of a prognostic model and the impact of mutations in patients with lower-risk myelodysplastic syndromes. J Clin Oncol 2012;30(27):3376–82.

37. Hoff FW, Madanat YF. Molecular drivers of myelodysplastic neoplasms (MDS)-classification and prognostic relevance. Cells 2023;12(4):627. https://doi.org/10.3390/cells12040627.

38. Papaemmanuil E, Gerstung M, Malcovati L, et al. Clinical and biological implications of driver mutations in myelodysplastic syndromes. Blood 2013;122(22): 3616–27 [quiz: 3699].

39. Haferlach T, Nagata Y, Grossmann V, et al. Landscape of genetic lesions in 944 patients with myelodysplastic syndromes. Leukemia 2014;28(2):241–7.

40. Sauta E, Robin M, Bersanelli M, et al. Real-world validation of molecular international prognostic scoring system for myelodysplastic syndromes. J Clin Oncol 2023;41(15):2827–42.

41. Madanat Y, Sekeres MA. Optimizing the use of hypomethylating agents in myelodysplastic syndromes: selecting the candidate, predicting the response, and enhancing the activity. Semin Hematol 2017;54(3):147–53.

42. Malcovati L, Papaemmanuil E, Bowen DT, et al. Clinical significance of SF3B1 mutations in myelodysplastic syndromes and myelodysplastic/myeloproliferative neoplasms. Blood 2011;118(24):6239–46.

43. Papaemmanuil E, Cazzola M, Boultwood J, et al. Somatic SF3B1 mutation in myelodysplasia with ring sideroblasts. N Engl J Med 2011;365(15):1384–95.

44. Visconte V, Rogers HJ, Singh J, et al. SF3B1 haploinsufficiency leads to formation of ring sideroblasts in myelodysplastic syndromes. Blood 2012;120(16):3173–86.

45. Malcovati L, Stevenson K, Papaemmanuil E, et al. SF3B1-mutant MDS as a distinct disease subtype: a proposal from the International Working Group for the Prognosis of MDS. Blood 2020;136(2):157–70.
46. Bejar R, Stevenson K, Abdel-Wahab O, et al. Clinical effect of point mutations in myelodysplastic syndromes. N Engl J Med 2011;364(26):2496–506.
47. Jadersten M, Saft L, Smith A, et al. TP53 mutations in low-risk myelodysplastic syndromes with del(5q) predict disease progression. J Clin Oncol 2011;29(15): 1971–9.
48. Della Porta MG, Galli A, Bacigalupo A, et al. Clinical effects of driver somatic mutations on the outcomes of patients with myelodysplastic syndromes treated with allogeneic hematopoietic stem-cell transplantation. J Clin Oncol 2016;34(30): 3627–37.
49. Haase D, Stevenson KE, Neuberg D, et al. TP53 mutation status divides myelodysplastic syndromes with complex karyotypes into distinct prognostic subgroups. Leukemia 2019;33(7):1747–58.
50. Farrukh F, Chetram D, Al-Kali A, et al. Real-world experience with luspatercept and predictors of response in myelodysplastic syndromes with ring sideroblasts. Am J Hematol 2022;97(6):E210–4.
51. Zeidan AM, Platzbecker U, Garcia-Manero G, et al. Longer-term benefit of luspatercept in transfusion-dependent lower-risk myelodysplastic syndromes with ring sideroblasts. Blood 2022;140(20):2170–4.
52. Platzbecker U, Gotze KS, Kiewe P, et al. Long-term efficacy and safety of luspatercept for anemia treatment in patients with lower-risk myelodysplastic syndromes: the phase II PACE-MDS study. J Clin Oncol 2022;40(33):3800–7.
53. Adema V, Khouri J, Ni Y, et al. Analysis of distinct SF3B1 hotspot mutations in relation to clinical phenotypes and response to therapy in myeloid neoplasia. Leuk Lymphoma 2021;62(3):735–8.
54. Seiler M, Yoshimi A, Darman R, et al. H3B-8800, an orally available small-molecule splicing modulator, induces lethality in spliceosome-mutant cancers. Nat Med 2018;24(4):497–504.
55. Steensma DP, Wermke M, Klimek VM, et al. Results of a clinical trial of H3B-8800, a splicing modulator, in patients with myelodysplastic syndromes (MDS), acute myeloid leukemia (AML) or chronic myelomonocytic leukemia (CMML). Blood 2019;134(Supplement_1):673.
56. DiNardo CD, Stein EM, de Botton S, et al. Durable remissions with ivosidenib in IDH1-mutated relapsed or refractory AML. N Engl J Med 2018;378(25):2386–98.
57. Sallman DA, Foran JM, Watts JM, et al. Ivosidenib in patients with IDH1-mutant relapsed/refractory myelodysplastic syndrome (R/R MDS): updated enrollment and results of a phase 1 dose-escalation and expansion substudy. J Clin Oncol 2022;40(16_suppl):7053.
58. Positive first trial of enasidenib for AML. Cancer Discov 2017;7(8):OF1.
59. DiNardo CD, Venugopal S, Lachowiez CA, et al. Targeted therapy with the mutant IDH2 inhibitor enasidenib for high-risk IDH2-mutant myelodysplastic syndrome. Blood Adv 2023;7(11):2378–87.
60. Watts JM, Baer MR, Yang J, et al. Olutasidenib alone or with azacitidine in IDH1-mutated acute myeloid leukaemia and myelodysplastic syndrome: phase 1 results of a phase 1/2 trial. Lancet Haematol 2023;10(1):e46–58.
61. de Botton S, Fenaux P, Yee KWL, et al. Olutasidenib (FT-2102) induces durable complete remissions in patients with relapsed or refractory IDH1-mutated AML. Blood Adv 2023;7(13):3117–27.

62. Huber S, Baer C, Hutter S, et al. AML and MDS classification according to Who 2022 and international consensus classification: do we invent a babylonian confusion of languages? Blood 2022;140(Supplement 1):555–6.

63. Mosquera Orgueira A, Perez Encinas M, Diaz Varela NA, et al. Supervised machine learning improves risk stratification in newly diagnosed myelodysplastic syndromes: an analysis of the Spanish group of myelodysplastic syndromes. Blood 2022;140(Supplement 1):1132–4.

64. Haferlach C, Huber S, Mueller H, et al. MDS classification - do we still have to count blasts? Blood 2022;140(Supplement 1):1130–1.

65. Fenaux P, Mufti GJ, Hellstrom-Lindberg E, et al. Efficacy of azacitidine compared with that of conventional care regimens in the treatment of higher-risk myelodysplastic syndromes: a randomised, open-label, phase III study. Lancet Oncol 2009;10(3):223–32.

66. Kantarjian H, Issa JP, Rosenfeld CS, et al. Decitabine improves patient outcomes in myelodysplastic syndromes: results of a phase III randomized study. Cancer 2006;106(8):1794–803.

67. Garcia-Manero G, Griffiths EA, Steensma DP, et al. Oral cedazuridine/decitabine for MDS and CMML: a phase 2 pharmacokinetic/pharmacodynamic randomized crossover study. Blood 2020;136(6):674–83.

68. Fenaux P, Santini V, Spiriti MAA, et al. A phase 3 randomized, placebo-controlled study assessing the efficacy and safety of epoetin-α in anemic patients with low-risk MDS. Leukemia 2018;32(12):2648–58.

69. Park S, Fenaux P, Greenberg P, et al. Efficacy and safety of darbepoetin alpha in patients with myelodysplastic syndromes: a systematic review and meta-analysis. Br J Haematol 2016;174(5):730–47.

70. Santini V, Almeida A, Giagounidis A, et al. Randomized phase III study of lenalidomide versus placebo in RBC transfusion-dependent patients with lower-risk non-del(5q) myelodysplastic syndromes and ineligible for or refractory to erythropoiesis-stimulating agents. J Clin Oncol 2016;34(25):2988–96.

71. Jabbour E, Short NJ, Montalban-Bravo G, et al. Randomized phase 2 study of low-dose decitabine vs low-dose azacitidine in lower-risk MDS and MDS/MPN. Blood 2017;130(13):1514–22.

UNITED STATES POSTAL SERVICE ® Statement of Ownership, Management, and Circulation (All Periodicals Publications Except Requester Publications)

1. Publication Title	2. Publication Number	3. Filing Date
CLINICS IN LABORATORY MEDICINE	000 – 713	9/18/2023

4. Issue Frequency	5. Number of Issues Published Annually	6. Annual Subscription Price
MAR, JUN, SEP, DEC	4	$291.00

7. Complete Mailing Address of Known Office of Publication (Not printer) (Street, city, county, state, and ZIP+4®)

ELSEVIER INC.
230 Park Avenue, Suite 800
New York, NY 10169

Contact Person
Malathi Samayan

Telephone (Include area code)
91-44-4299-4507

8. Complete Mailing Address of Headquarters or General Business Office of Publisher (Not printer)

ELSEVIER INC.
230 Park Avenue, Suite 800
New York, NY 10169

9. Full Names and Complete Mailing Addresses of Publisher, Editor, and Managing Editor (Do not leave blank)

Publisher (Name and complete mailing address)

Dolores Meloni, ELSEVIER INC.
1600 JOHN F KENNEDY BLVD. SUITE 1600
PHILADELPHIA, PA 19103-2899

Editor (Name and complete mailing address)

TAYLOR HAYES, ELSEVIER INC.
1600 JOHN F KENNEDY BLVD. SUITE 1600
PHILADELPHIA, PA 19103-2899

Managing Editor (Name and complete mailing address)

PATRICK MANLEY, ELSEVIER INC.
1600 JOHN F KENNEDY BLVD. SUITE 1600
PHILADELPHIA, PA 19103-2899

10. Owner (Do not leave blank. If the publication is owned by a corporation, give the name and address of the corporation immediately followed by the names and addresses of all stockholders owning or holding 1 percent or more of the total amount of stock. If not owned by a corporation, give the names and addresses of the individual owners. If owned by a partnership or other unincorporated firm, give its name and address as well as those of each individual owner. If the publication is published by a nonprofit organization, give its name and address.)

Full Name	Complete Mailing Address
WHOLLY OWNED SUBSIDIARY OF REED/ELSEVIER, US HOLDINGS	1600 JOHN F KENNEDY BLVD. SUITE 1600 PHILADELPHIA, PA 19103-2899

11. Known Bondholders, Mortgagees, and Other Security Holders Owning or Holding 1 Percent or More of Total Amount of Bonds, Mortgages, or Other Securities. If none, check box ▶ ☐ None

Full Name	Complete Mailing Address
N/A	

12. Tax Status (For completion by nonprofit organizations authorized to mail at nonprofit rates) (Check one)
The purpose, function, and nonprofit status of this organization and the exempt status for federal income tax purposes:
☒ Has Not Changed During Preceding 12 Months
☐ Has Changed During Preceding 12 Months (Publisher must submit explanation of change with this statement)

PS Form 3526, July 2014 [Page 1 of 4 (see instructions page 4)] PSN: 7530-01-000-9931   PRIVACY NOTICE: See our privacy policy on www.usps.com.

---

13. Publication Title	14. Issue Date for Circulation Data Below
CLINICS IN LABORATORY MEDICINE	JULY 2023

15. Extent and Nature of Circulation			Average No. Copies Each Issue During Preceding 12 Months	No. Copies of Single Issue Published Nearest to Filing Date
a. Total Number of Copies (Net press run)			59	60
b. Paid Circulation (By Mail and Outside the Mail)	(1)	Mailed Outside-County Paid Subscriptions Stated on PS Form 3541 (Include paid distribution above nominal rate, advertiser's proof copies, and exchange copies)	35	39
	(2)	Mailed In-County Paid Subscriptions Stated on PS Form 3541 (Include paid distribution above nominal rate, advertiser's proof copies, and exchange copies)	0	0
	(3)	Paid Distribution Outside the Mails Including Sales Through Dealers and Carriers, Street Vendors, Counter Sales, and Other Paid Distribution Outside USPS®	12	9
	(4)	Paid Distribution by Other Classes of Mail Through the USPS (e.g., First-Class Mail®)	6	6
c. Total Paid Distribution [Sum of 15b (1), (2), (3), and (4)]		▶	53	54
d. Free or Nominal Rate Distribution (By Mail and Outside the Mail)	(1)	Free or Nominal Rate Outside-County Copies included on PS Form 3541	5	5
	(2)	Free or Nominal Rate In-County Copies Included on PS Form 3541	0	0
	(3)	Free or Nominal Rate Copies Mailed at Other Classes Through the USPS (e.g., First-Class Mail)	0	0
	(4)	Free or Nominal Rate Distribution Outside the Mail (Carriers or other means)	1	1
e. Total Free or Nominal Rate Distribution (Sum of 15d (1), (2), (3) and (4))		▶	6	6
f. Total Distribution (Sum of 15c and 15e)		▶	59	60
g. Copies not Distributed (See Instructions to Publishers #4 (page #3))		▶	0	0
h. Total (Sum of 15f and g)		▶	59	60
i. Percent Paid (15c divided by 15f times 100)		▶	89.53%	90%

* If you are claiming electronic copies, go to line 16 on page 3. If you are not claiming electronic copies, skip to line 17 on page 3.

PS Form 3526, July 2014 (Page 2 of 4)

16. Electronic Copy Circulation		Average No. Copies Each Issue During Preceding 12 Months	No. Copies of Single Issue Published Nearest to Filing Date
a. Paid Electronic Copies	▶		
b. Total Paid Print Copies (Line 15c) + Paid Electronic Copies (Line 16a)	▶		
c. Total Print Distribution (Line 15f) + Paid Electronic Copies (Line 16a)	▶		
d. Percent Paid (Both Print & Electronic Copies) (16b divided by 16c × 100)	▶		

☒ I certify that 50% of all my distributed copies (electronic and print) are paid above a nominal price.

17. Publication of Statement of Ownership

☒ If the publication is a general publication, publication of this statement is required. Will be printed in the DECEMBER 2023 issue of this publication.   ☐ Publication not required.

18. Signature and Title of Editor, Publisher, Business Manager, or Owner	Date
Malathi Samayan Malathi Samayan - Distribution Controller	9/18/2023

I certify that all information furnished on this form is true and complete. I understand that anyone who furnishes false or misleading information on this form or who omits material or information requested on the form may be subject to criminal sanctions (including fines and imprisonment) and/or civil sanctions (including civil penalties).

PS Form 3526, July 2014 (Page 3 of 4)   PRIVACY NOTICE: See our privacy policy on www.usps.com

Moving?

Make sure your subscription moves with you!

To notify us of your new address, find your **Clinics Account Number** (located on your mailing label above your name), and contact customer service at:

Email: journalscustomerservice-usa@elsevier.com

800-654-2452 (subscribers in the U.S. & Canada)
314-447-8871 (subscribers outside of the U.S. & Canada)

Fax number: 314-447-8029

Elsevier Health Sciences Division
Subscription Customer Service
3251 Riverport Lane
Maryland Heights, MO 63043

*To ensure uninterrupted delivery of your subscription, please notify us at least 4 weeks in advance of move.

Printed and bound by CPI Group (UK) Ltd, Croydon, CR0 4YY

03/10/2024

01040469-0020